Proceedings and Collections
Anti-cancer, anti-cancer metastasis research

THE NARRATE OF INNOVATION THEORIES

and

METHODS OF CANCER TREATMENT VOLUME 1

Reform • Innovation • Development

The promising prospects of Immunomodulating drugs

Authors: Bin Wu and Lily Xu
Editors: Bin Wu and Lily Xu
Translators: Bin Wu and Lily Xu

authorHOUSE

AuthorHouse™
1663 Liberty Drive
Bloomington, IN 47403
www.authorhouse.com
Phone: 833-262-8899

Published by AuthorHouse 10/07/2021

ISBN: 978-1-6655-3032-3 (sc)
ISBN: 978-1-6655-3033-0 (e)

Library of Congress Control Number: 2021913205

Print information available on the last page.

This book is printed on acid-free paper.

The human body is a hero.
All healing of the human body is an innate self healing
and is an inherent biological process.
Our health is controlled by our hands.
We are the drivers for our health.

The doctors are at their best with modifying, regulating, controlling the circumstances, the conditions under which we live, such as what type of diet, how much rest we have, how mch food we take, how much sleep we have, how much exercise we have, how much worry not justified, how much anxiety not justified.

It is very important in our lifes to stay in the present time, the present is a gift.
This is the way we should think of and this is the way we should live.

The main purpose for us to be healthy, it is that where we have the state of functional excellence which allow us to get the best mentally and physically and spiritually for ourselves (our organisum or our bodies).

<u>The cancer cure should be through regulation and controlling rather than killing</u>

In this book, I summary the new things and our past work together in the detail, <u>especially emphazie the medications for cancer treatment.</u>

Life is precious and let us prevent from cancer and other diseases.

Let us learn the things through hard work and others wisdom.

THE IMPORTANT CONCEPT OF CANCER TREATMENT

The cancer cure should be through regulation and control rather than killing.

Healing should be through regulation and control rather than killing.

The last step in curing cancer is to mobilize the reappearance of the host's control, rather than destroy the last cancer cells.

Cancer prevention is the same important as cancer treatment.

In another word, keeping our bodied healthy immune function is essential for completely curing cancer.

For the aboving concepts, there are some experiments to support them as the followings in brief:

From the father of medicine Hippocrates, "Everyone has a physician inside him or her; we just have to help it in its work. The natural healing force within each one of us is the greatest force in getting well. The next questions:

How can we wake up widely our inside physician?

Now along the technological rapid development, our human being works very hard to search for the good ways to live longer and to keep diseases free such as fasting, medication, meditation etc.

From Chinese book **"Huang Di Nei Jing"**, it is also said, *"the disease is not the inherent part of human body, which can be gained and also can be removed. If it can not be removed, it is because the method is not found.*

This means, the health is our normal state. If any disease happens to us, we should or could find the correct way to remove it. Our inherent part is health.

From Shong Han Theory, it is said, "*losing grain can cure the diseases*".

With thousand years people work hard to search for the ways for curing the diseases.

Where is the way for cancer theory?
How can it make cancer free from us?
How can we remove the cancer fear from us?

During our experiments, we surprisely found that cancer can disappear by their own or even if the cancer cells are injected into the body, the cancer will not grow at all.

Here some example of our experiments which were done as the following in brief, the detail and more experiment will be explained in detail in this book chapters:

1. From experimental studies, the process of cancer cell metastasis in the lymphatic tract was observed:

A. After transplanting 1×10^6 cancer cells under the skin of the inner side of the mouse paw pads, the animals were sacrificed at different times for local lymph node histological observation.

One hour after the transplantation of tumor cells, a single cancer cell was found in the marginal sinus of the cochineal lymph node, but no mitotic phase was seen;

After 3 hours, there are 3-5 groups of tumor cells in the marginal sinus of the cochineal lymph node, and mitotic phases can be seen;

After 5 hours, there are piles of cancer cells in the marginal sinus of the rouge lymph node, and some tumor cells have entered the middle sinus.

Twenty-four hours later, metastases had formed in the rouge lymph nodes. Scattered cancer cells were found in the middle sinus.

After 3-5 days, the popliteal lymph nodes have been occupied by metastatic tumor cells, and tumor cells and metastatic lesions were found in the second and third lymph nodes near the iliac artery and renal hilum.

Generally, metastases can be found in multiple lymph nodes after 3 days. Some cancer cells (such as Ehrlich's ascites carcinoma) form metastases only 5 days, and the metastases of rouge fossa lymph nodes can undergo degeneration and necrosis, and lymph node immune cells proliferate.

However, after 10 days, no cancer cells were found in the lymph nodes, and they were eventually destroyed by the host cells and disappeared.

The above experimental results suggest:

5 days after Ehrlich ascites cancer cells form metastases, the rouge lymph nodes may **undergo degeneration and necrosis**.

It indicates that the lymph node itself is a peripheral immune organ, which should be monitored and swallowed by cancer cells.

After 10 days, no cancer cells were found in the lymph nodes, which were obviously eliminated by the host's immune cells.

It is suggested that the treatment of anti-cancer metastasis can use the anti-cancer system and anti-cancer factors to protect and activate the host to destroy the invading cancer cells. The immune defense in the body can remove the cancer cells completely.

B. *Carry out experimental research on tumors and create cancer-bearing animal models*

A sterile tumor specimen was removed from the clinical operating table, and it was transplanted into experimental animals after 0.5h of warm ischemia. It was done more than 100 times (400 animals) without success. There was no any single animal which grew cancer yet.

However, when the thymus was first removed and then the cancer cells were transplanted in some mice, the cancer cells grew in the mice, which means after the removal of the main immune organ Thymus, it can promote the cancer cell growth. And this experiment was successful in the 210 animals.

Some injections of cortisone can reduce the immunity of mice and it can also promote the cancer cell growth so that the cancer cells can be transplanted successfully to the mice.

5 days after the thymus is cut and the cancer cells were transplanted, the large soybean nodules can grow after 5-6 days, and they grew to a large tumor of the thumb in 10-21 days.

Transplanted cancer can survive for 3-4 weeks, but it cannot be passed down to generations.

1. *Through this study, it is found that removal of the thymus can create a cancer-bearing animal model, and injection of cortisone can also help create a cancer-bearing animal model.*

2. *Research conclusions prove that the occurrence and development of cancer are related to the host's body immunity, and have a very obvious relationship with immune organs and immune organ tissue functions.*

3. *The results of this study confirmed that the immune organ thymus (Thymus, Th) and immune function have an extremely definite relationship with the occurrence and development of cancer.*

If the host Thymus is removed, it may be made into a cancer-bearing animal model, and if it is not removed, it cannot be a cancer-bearing animal model.

Injecting immunosuppressive drugs to reduce host immunity function will help create cancer-bearing animal models. Without injections of immuno-lowering drugs, cancer-bearing animal models cannot be created.

This result shows that immune organs and immunity are negatively correlated with cancer cell growth (during the cancer transplantation experiment and cancer implanation experiment) into solid cancer.

With immunodeficiency or reduced immunity, cancer cells of transplantation can implant and grow tumors without being swallowed or destroyed or damaged by the host's immune cells.

C. **From the animal experiments, cancer cells S_{180} 1×10^6** were injected into Kuanming mouse through the tail vein, which were eliminated by 99% after 24-36 hours, and only less than 0.1 of cancer cells can be survived and can be grown and form the metastasis.

Who destroyed these 99% cancer cells?

It suggested that some of cancer cells were destroyed by the uncomfortable environment or the crash force or obstracting in the circulation of blood, however the most of the cancer cells after entering into the blood circulation mainly be destroyed by the host immune defences system such as the immune cells.

Hence, it should protect the host immune sysmentand should activate the host immune system function during treating the cancer and should not strike the host immune system and should not decreasethe host immune defense function.

In this book, there are many ways which are provided to protect the host immune functions.

In brief, healing is a biological process and is innate. Our body is the hero. There is no such things as chemicals, drugs, food and other ingredient that will take place of the living process of life.

All healing is self healing. Healing is not something that somebody else does to you. Healing is something you do for yourself.

The miracle is the living process and is it-self but what the doctor can do is the doctor can make decision about lifestyle which can enhance the person life or destroy the person life.

The choice or general speaking is yours and you have to make these decisions.

This is a book of the summary and reflection of the part of the past work for the cancer theorepy.

The extremely important concepts of cancer prevention:

1. _Cancer is a disease that can **be prevented**_ because now sinscien already proved that more than 90% of cancer occurrence are related to the environmental factors such as air, water, food, soil, and the social environment, etc.

2. Cancer is a diseae that threatens the human life so that the human _**should prevent and treat cancer**_; meanwhile it should realize that cancer can be prevented and cured; also it is very important to realize _**that cancer prevention should be put on the same attention and the same level at the same time**_ in order to stop and to eliminate the cancer occurrence at its source and before cancer happens.

3. _**It should do three early things: the early discovery, the early diagnosis, the early treatment. Cancer can be cured**_.

TABLE OF CONTENTS

TO ALL MY READERS

First, I deeply appreciate you for taking your precious time to open this book about the wellness of human beings.

Why do cancer and metastasis happen?
How should we treat it?
Can it be reversed by our bodies?
Can cancer be reversed and, if so, how?

During our experiments, some of the cancer in the rats disappeared after the cancer cells already moved to lymph nodes on the day of 8. When we injected cancer cells into mice and the lymph nodes had necrosis, eventually, the cancer disappeared.

All of these proved that our bodies had the ability to eliminate the cancer cells during our repeated experiments.

How can we help our bodies activate or enhance these abilities to remove cancer cells?
How can our body's physician be woken up to remove all cancer cells?

Technology has been dramatically developed, and many mysteries in the past have been clearly explained by scientific evidence. Many chronic diseases such as heart disease, cancer, metabolic diseases, and diabetics can be prevented and cured.

Cancer prevention is as important as the cancer treatment (it must be emphasized that prevention and treatment need the same attention and the same lever at the same time).

This book mainly emphasizes the medications which we use for treating cancer patients, especially the immunotherapy medications (the drugs' mechanism, the experiments, and the clinical verifications, etc).

In this book, many basic and clinical experiments in the lab proved and provided that cancer treatment should be through controlling it and should regulate the recovery of the body's ability of controlling the cancer, not through killing the final cancer cell. These experiments proved many of the new and important theories, such as:

The leading or guiding ideas of the new cancer model are:

Regulation and signal transmission between cells in cancer patients are disrupted rather than lost; the carcinogenesis is considered to be a *continuum with the possibility of reversal*.

Or it is considered that carcinogenesis is a continuum with the **possibility of reversal.**

Our body is constantly changing all the time and today's you is different from tomorrow's you.

Let us gather our knowledge:

1. *When I reviewed Greek medicine, the words from the father of medicine, Hippocrates gave me great relevance about our health:*

"Everyone has a physician inside him or her; we just have to help it in its work. The natural healing force within each one of us is the greatest force in getting well. Our food should be our medicine. Our medicine should be our food. But to eat when you are sick is to feed your sickness."

- Hippocrates

This means our body has infinite healing wisdom.

How can we wake up completely this inner physician or search out this inside physician to get complete recovery?

In this book, we have written down some of this wisdom in detail, with some of the experiments in medication (the evidence), methods for cancer treatment, etc., which it can benefit our human health.

In this book, there are many medications which were tested and verified, and they had excellent effects on cancer patients.

Of course, there are many other ways such as fasting, exercise, meditation, etc.

2. *Technology has rapidly developed.*

Many things which we once thought of as impossible have now been achieved.

The understanding of life, such as physiology, pathogenetic pathophysiology, genetics, etc. grows fast as new technology and science develops rapidly after the knowledge and findings of humans increase.

Many mysteries of the living body have been explained and verified or confirmed by facts, such as:

1) Some cardiovascular diseases can be reversed, and *nitric oxide*, especially the **endothelium cell** is important for the vascular system to function well (1).

It was found that good circulation is the key for our health, such as cancer metastasis and for our immune system (. As Dr. William Osler said: we are as old as our arteries.

2) Hyperinsulinemia (insulin resistance) and high carbohydrates are related to many diseases, such as diabetes (diabetes can be reversed completely), to the fibroid and to prostate diseases (2, 3, 4)

3) Our body can recycle to keep healthy, which is good for aging and many other diseases. It also has proven the concepts for many disease treatments, for a variety of diseases, which comes from the Nobel Prize in Physiology or Medicine 2016, awarded to Yoshinori Ohsumi "for his discoveries of mechanisms for autophagy." The concept gave evidence for fasting therapy for many diseases, such as aging, diabetics, cancer, and others more.

4) Our endocrine system is extremely important and related to many cancers and other diseases, such as estrogen (it is clear to relate this with breast cancer and other cancers, but especially those found in women), testosterone (it is one of the factors which is related to prostate cancer growth), *insulin (which is related to many conditions of the body)*, etc.

The human being is evolving and is now a hormonally modified human being. It is very important to keep the hormone balance between catabolism and anabolism, mainly by insulin (from the pancreas) and other hormones.

Our daily habits change our hormone levels so that if we change our habits, we can control our hormone balance to control our health situation. We will become the drivers for our health.

In addition, Hippocrates, the father of Western **medicine**, believed **fasting** enabled the body to heal itself. (He believed in the infinite healing wisdom inside human beings).

Paracelsus, another great healer in the Western tradition, wrote 500 years ago that "**fasting** is the greatest remedy, the physician within."

In brief, lifestyle changes are extremely important for our health, our aging, and our mind. This discipline is extremely important to keep good health.

3. *In Chinese <<Huangdi neijing>>, there were:*

The disease is not the thing belonging to our bodies, which can come and can be removed. If the disease cannot be removed, it is because the correct methods have not been found.

Persistence, persistence, and persistence!

During the time of COVID-19, I have stayed at home reviewing many medical textbooks about anatomy, biochemistry, immunology as well as clinical and experimental research data. One lecture I listened to repeatedly was given by a surgeon. One phrase that stuck out to me was, "Perhaps brains are important, but nothing and nothing is as important as persistence, persistence, and persistence.

"The road of science is not smooth, and similarly, neither is the road of life. After a long, challenging, and tearing road, this is finally here now."

How is this book new and what is it about?

This book focuses on cancer prevention and treatment, specifically on immune pharmacy.

We must accept the factors:

Technology is developing dramatically; the wonders of modern technology make many mysteries clear and clinical data has shown that many diseases can be cured and prevented by lifestyle changes and by our inside systems.

However, cancer is still a dangerous disease that threatens many people's wellbeing.

How can we help control these diseases?

What is the road that can cure and prevent these diseases?

This book will discuss a new way of controlling and preventing cancer. I hope you enjoy reading.

References:

(1). Prevent and Reverse Heart Disease: The Revolutionary, Scientifically Proven, Nutrition-Based Cure, by Caldwell B. Esselstyn Jr. Publisher : Avery; 1ˢᵗ edition (January 31, 2008)

(2). Hyperinsulinemia: An Early Indicator of Metabolic Dysfunction, Dylan D Thomas, Barbara E Corkey, Nawfal W Istfan, Caroline M Apovian.
Journal of the Endocrine Society, Volume 3, Issue 9, September 2019, Pages 1727–1747, https://doi.org/10.1210/js.2019-00065

(3). Diet-Induced Hyperinsulinemia as a Key Factor in the Etiology of Both Benign Prostatic Hyperplasia and Essential Hypertension?
Wolfgang Kopp, Mariatrosterstrasse 41, 8043 Graz, Austria.
Nutr Metab Insights. 2018; 11: 1178638818773072. Published online 2018 May 8. doi: 10.1177/1178638818773072 PMCID: PMC6238249 PMID: 30455570

(4). Uterine Leiomyomata in Relation to Insulin-Like Growth Factor-I, Insulin, and Diabetes.
Donna Day Baird,1 Greg Travlos,2 Ralph Wilson,2 David B Dunson,3 Michael C Hill,4 Aimee A D'Aloisio,1 Stephanie J London,1 and Joel M Schectman5
Published in final edited form as: Epidemiology. 2009 Jul; 20(4): 604–610. PMC2856640 PMID: 19305350

(5). International narcotics control board for 2009. New York: United Nations, 2010). Canadian Gazette. Controlled Drugs and Substances Ac

(6). The book<< new concept and new ways of treatment of cancer metastasis>>. Xu Ze, etc. Pressed in 2016 by authorhouse Inc. U.SA

Bin Wu, Lily Xu
04-27-21, in Timonium, Maryland USA

ABOUT THE AUTHOR 1

**A brief introduction to the first author
and the main translator and the editor**

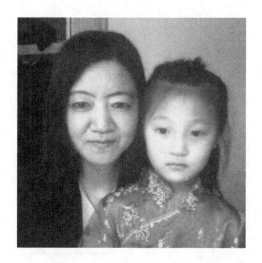

Bin Wu, MD, Ph.D., graduated from College of Yunyang of Tongji University of Medical Sciences for her MD degree; Studied her Master degree and her Ph. D degree in Sun Yat-Sen University of Medical Sciences. After she received her Ph.D., she worked as a Post-doctoral fellow in the Johns Hopkins Medical School and University of Maryland Medical School. She passed all of her USMLE tests and is going to do her residency training in America. She dedicated herself to oncology clinical and research. Her goal is to conquer cancer, which she believes this great contribution to our health. She has a daughter, named Lily Xu who gives great help with writing and editing and drawing all of the pictures in the books.

ABOUT THE AUTHOR 2

**A Brief introduction to the second author and
the editor and my only trustful advisor**

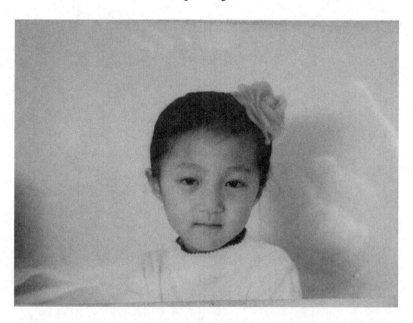

Lily Xu was born on November 17th 2006 and is in Advanced Biology Class in the high school since 2020. In 2020, she won the Robot designing model in Maryland and Math Model in Baltimore County in Maryland and she is in the Baltimore country honor banding. She helps with this book edition and others. She had an art presented in the Walter Art Museum in Baltimore at the age of 6; she got the fourth place trophy in the ES Double Digits or 24 and 24 games in the Baltimore County in Maryland; she got the first trophy in the BCPS STEM FAIR PHYSICS in Baltimore County; when she was in the sixth grade, she passed the advanced Math for 7th grade(which means the 8th grade math) test and moved the 8th grade math class and now she takes high school Math class; she loves the reading and the writing and she finished many seires of books and in 2019 summary she start to do volunteer job in the publish libarary. She got $9000 scholarship award for the Peabody music program in the Johns Hopkins University. She edits all of my books for the publishing and drew all of the pictures in this book. In 2018 and 2019 she was chosen into Baltimore county Middle school Honor Band. In 2018 the robotic team which she attended for years got designing-award from the Baltimore county so that this robotic team came to Maryland State for the Robotic contest in 2019. On January 19th, 2019 she got the Robotic designing award in Maryland. She edits all of my books for the publishing and drew all of the pictures in the book. In 2019 she was chosen by Baltimore County for one duel and one ensemble to play Clarion. Now she is in the nineth grade for her high school and while she was chosen to attend of Maryland state debate team in March 2021. She loves study and challenge and has execellent judgement. In 2021, she already won four medals for the different contests.

PREFACE

This monographs is not only written with a pen, *but also made with real and hard work or done with actually working or performing.*

The contents of these monographs all come from clinical practice experience and lessons, review, reflection, and **practice produces the reality and practice leads to know the truth**.

The contents of these monographs are all derived from the experimental research results of their own laboratories, and **the experiments produced results or achievement.**

The content of these monographs is a true record of scientific thinking and scientific practice from experiment to clinical, and then from clinical to experimental. The summary of experimental research and clinical verification data has risen to the essence of theory; meanwhile the new discoveries, new understandings, and new theories have been proposed. **All of these innovative theories of clinical practicability can be used to guide clinical treatment**.

All should be converted to clinical applications through translational medicine to guide clinical treatment and benefit patients.

The contents of these monographs:

They are all their own more than half a century of therapeutic practice experience and 30 years of experimental research materials. They are summarized, organized, and compiled into this book. The scientific research results and scientific and technological innovation series **are all their own materials, and some of them are international firsts. All of them are the original innovation. Some are internationally advanced and independent innovations, all with independent intellectual property rights.**

The content of this series of monographs:

Fully or completely is in line with or corresponds to the content of translational medicine.

Our 28-year scientific research route has been from clinical to experimental, clinical and experimental, and returns to the clinical to solve clinical practical problems. Our research model is completely in line with or matches this new medical research model.

Translational or transformation Medicine

Transformation Medicine recently develops rapidly and vigorously internationally.

This new medical research model advocates patient-centered, discovering and asking questions from clinical work, conducting in-depth basic research, and then quickly turning basic research results into clinical applications to improve the overall level of medical care and ultimately benefit patients.

Academician Chen Zhu, the former minister of the Ministry of Health, has analyzed the connotation of translational medicine:

First, translational medicine is a science that passes **through a two-way channel from laboratory to clinic and from clinical to laboratory for In-depth understanding the mechanisms of the occurrence and development of diseases and mechanisms of health protection promotion, and exploring new prevention and control strategies.**

Second, we **must transform scientific research results into clinical, public health, practical, interventional methods, technologies, and programs for their popularization.**

The World Health Organization proposes that medicine in the 21st century should not continue to use disease as the main research field, but should take human health as the main research direction.

Academician Chen Zhu pointed out:

The health service model should be transformed. It is necessary to shift from treatment-oriented in the late stage of serious diseases to prevention-oriented, and move the gate forward and sink the center of gravity. Strengthening research

in preventive medicine is a major issue in my country and the transformation of the global medical model.

The focus of my country's translational or transformation medicine research, the modernization and internationalization of Chinese medicine and Chinese medication is one of the key contents of my country's translational medicine research.

ACKNOWLEDGEMENTS

When I was close to finish this book, I recalled my parents dramatically because I realized their words and behavour and spirit are so useful for me to live well. I looked at my parents and my childhood pictures and many beautiful momery showed up. I learned things from my parents. Now I realize that my father was such an excellent person on the healthy skills and the wisest doctor in my mind. He realized that the lifestyle of an individual is such an important thing for preventing and curing a disease. I learn to have a strong will.

If they were still alive, I would understand more medicine and do more things for others because I would get more things from their experience.

I thank my parents to enlighten me about the medicine since I started to understand things. My parents want me to do more contribution our societies.

When I was at the very young age, my father told me **how the bone morrow is important**. At that time, I didn't understand anything about immune system. My mother always told me something such **as garlic, ginger** function and why we eat them while I watched her cooked the dishes.

I thank my parents for trying very hard to lead me like to become a medical professional because both of them really loved what they dedicate and they wanted me to follow their footsteps. Both them let me come to the operation room to shadow them even far before I went to medical school. My father was excellent on many medical things. I miss my parents.

In addition, I **thank for Lily Xu who helps me editing all of my work and always give me the great and crystal idea and suggestion. She told me that the grammar should be paid attention to.** Thank for she studied hard by her own so that I can concentrate on this book.

Second, this book is for all of people who concern human being health.

We are deep grateful to all of people who like our new ways to improve our human being health. I appreciate to anyone who encourages me to continue working on my career. I thank for any good word which is encouraging me.

My daughter Lily Xu gives me many smart and creative ideas while we were finishing this book. **The characteristics of she loves the challenge** and her judgment always encourages me to continue working hard to move on. I learn the new things from her daily. I have to admit she is really smart on thinking things.

I would like to express our sincere gratitude to the following:

1. All of Authorhouse staffs

2. Dr. Xu Ze and other workers who were involved in cancer patient care.

3. Mrs. Bo Wu's family and Mrs. Tao Wu's famly

4. I deeply thank my only daughter Lily Xu, for her help with me and for her wisdom, for <u>her understanding me</u> and <u>for her update knowledge and for her loving learning</u>.

Bin Wu, M.D., Ph.D
04-29-2021 in Timonium, Maryland in USA

This book is the summary and collections of the part of the past work.

1. **The important concept _of cancer treatment_:**

   <u>**The cancer cure should be through regulation and control rather than killing.**</u>

   Healing should be through regulation and control rather than killing.

   **The last step in curing cancer is to mobilize the reappearance of the host's control,** rather than destroy the last cancer cells.

   <u>_In another word, keeping our bodied healthy immune function is essential for completely curing cancer._</u>

2. **The important concept _of cancer prevention_:**

Cancer prevention is the same importance as cancer treatment. It should put on the same attention and the same level at the same time. It is very important to do three early things: the early discovery, the early diagnosis, the early treatment so that cure can be cured.

For the aboving concepts, we have some experients to support them in the following book content in the details.

Part I

**Scientific and technological innovation
Scientific research achievement**

The research on XZ-C immunomodulation anti-cancer traditional Chinese medication

The collections of scientific research achievements, scientific and technological innovation

Where is the way to conquer and defeat cancer? Or in order to win cancer, where is the road?

XUZE believes that the road is in scientific research------the road is in scientific research on the <u>prevention and treatment</u> of cancer, and the road is under the guidance of the scientific development concept.

Science----

is the endless frontier, our scientific research work has always followed the scientific development concept, based on known medicine, facing the future medicine, emerging disciplines, marginal disciplines, interdisciplinary disciplines or cross-disciplines;

is based on known science, explore future science and unknown knowledge;

is looking forward, after calming down and long-term hard work, and practicing the scientific development concept.

On the road of science, it is difficult to make strides, one scientific research step at a time, or step by step in scientific research;

on the road of science, it is facing the frontiers of science, striving for innovation and progress, adding bricks and tiles to the scientific research palace or research hall for conquering cancer.

Strive to take the innovative path of anti-cancer metastasis with Chinese characteristics or efforts to take the innovative way of China's characteristic anti-cancer metastasis

Take the road of modernization of Chinese medicine, promote the integration of Chinese medicine and Western medicine at the molecular level, and integrate with international medical modernization

TABLE OF CONTENTS

FOREWORD

Gratifying or Improving prospects for immunomodulatory drugs

No matter how complicated the mechanism behind cancer is, the body's immune suppression is the key to cancer progression.

Removal of immunosuppressive factors and restoration of system cells' recognition of cancer cells <u>can effectively defeat or resist cancer</u>. More and more research evidence shows that by regulating the body's immune system, it is possible to achieve the purpose of controlling cancer. The treatment of tumors by activating the body's anti-tumor immune system is currently an exciting area for researchers. The next major breakthrough in cancer is likely to come from this.

<u>*In order to discuss the etiology, pathogenesis, and pathophysiology of cancer, we conducted a series of animal experimental studies. From the analysis of experimental results, we have obtained the new discoveries and new enlightenments:*</u>

<u>*Atrophy of the thymus and low or decreasing immune function are one of the causes and pathogenesis of cancer. Therefore, Professor Xu Ze proposed at the international conference that one of the causes and pathogenesis of cancer may be atrophy of the thymus and impaired function of the central immune organs, immune function decreasing, immune surveillance ability reducing and immune escape.*</u>

As a result of laboratory experiments, it was found that:

The thymus of cancer-bearing mice showed progressive atrophy. The function of the central immune organ is impaired, the immune function is reduced, and the immune surveillance is low, <u>*so the treatment principle must be to prevent the thymus from progressive atrophy, to promote thymus hyperplasia, to protect the bone marrow hematopoietic function and to improve immune surveillance, which provides a theoretical basis and experimental basis for treatment of cancer with immune regulation and control.*</u>

5

Based on the enlightenment of the above experimental results on cancer etiology and pathogenesis, the new concepts and methods of XZ-C immunomodulatory therapy are proposed.

After 16 years of clinical examination and observation of more than 12,000 middle-stage and advanced-stage cancer patients in the oncology clinic, *it has been confirmed that the treatment principle of Thymus protection and enhancing immune function is reasonable and the efficacy is satisfactory.*

The application of immunomodulatory Chinese medicine has achieved good results, improved the quality of life, and significantly prolonged the survival period.

The XZ-C (XU ZE-China) immunomodulation method was first proposed by Professor Xu Ze in his book "New Concepts and Methods of Cancer Metastasis Treatment" in 2006.

He believes that **under normal circumstances, the cancer and the body's defenses are in a dynamic balance, and the occurrence of cancer is caused by the imbalance of the dynamic balance.** If the disordered state is adjusted to a normal level, the growth of cancer can be controlled and resolved, or if it is to adjust the disordered state to a normal level, it can control the growth of cancer and make cancer fade.

As we all know, the occurrence, development and prognosis of cancer are determined by the comparison of two factors, that is, the biological characteristics of cancer cells and the host body's own defense ability to restrict and defend against cancer cells. If the two are balanced, the cancer can be controlled; if the two are out of balance, the cancer will develop.

Under normal circumstances, the host's body itself has certain restrictions on cancer cells, but when the host's body is suffering from cancer, these restrictions and defense capabilities are inhibited and damaged to varying degrees, resulting in cancer cells losing immune surveillance and cancer cell immune escape so that cancer cells can further develop and metastasize.

Through the above 4 years of basic experimental research on the mechanism of recurrence and metastasis. After another 3 years of the tumor-inhibiting test in cancer-bearing mice from the internal experiment of natural medicine and herbal medicine. A batch of Chinese medicines with good tumor suppression rate were selected from Chinese herbal medicines to form XZ-C $_{1-10}$ anti-cancer immune-modulating Chinese medicine.

1

Overview and the experiments of the selection of the anti-cancer medications

A. _XZ-C immunomodulatory anti-cancer Chinese medications are the Chinese herbal medications which 48 kinds of Chinese herbal medicines with good tumor inhibition rate were selected and screened out from traditional Chinese herbal medicines through the tumor-bearing experiment of tumor-bearing mice in vivo performed._

After they were comprised or compounded into the compound, it showed that the tumor-inhibition rate of the compound was far greater than that of single drugs rate during the anti-tumor experiment in cancer-bearing mice.

_XZ-C$_1$ and XZ-C$_4$ are composed of 28 Chinese herbal medicines such as Shencao, Longyacao, and Shuyangquan. Among them, XZ-C$_{1-A}$ and XZ-C$_{1-B}$ 100% inhibit cancer cells, and 100% do not kill normal cells._

They have the function of supporting the rightness, strengthening the body, improving the body's immune function.

From our experiments, the results of XZ-C pharmacodynamic studies prove:

1) _It has a good tumor suppression rate for Ehrlich ascites carcinoma, S$_{180}$ and H$_{22}$ hepatocellular carcinoma;_

2) _it has a significant synergistic effects and attenuating toxic effects;_

3) _The experiment also proves that xz-c immune regulation and control Chinese medicine can significantly improve the immune function of human body._

XZ-C has the following unique characters:

1. *After acute toxicity experiments in mice, there were no obvious toxic and side effects;*

2. *There were no obvious toxic and side effects in the clinical long-term oral administration for several years (8-10 years).*

3. Oral administration of XZ-C immunomodulatory Chinese medicine during chemotherapy can significantly reduce side effects.

4. Oral administration of XZ-C medicine during chemotherapy intermittent period can increase white blood cells and increase hemoglobin.

5. 5. Most patients with advanced cancer are debilitating, fatigued, and lack of appetite. After taking XZ-C anti-cancer Chinese medicine for 4-8--12 weeks, they can significantly improve the appetite and sleep, relieve pain, and gradually restore physical strength.

B. *The Experimental Study of Fuzheng Peiben on Tumor-inhibiting and Immunity-enhancing Effects of S_{180}-bearing Mice*

1. The Purpose of the Experiement

Through more than decades of research and practice in the prevention and treatment of malignant tumors with integrated Chinese and Western medicine in my country, it has been found that many Chinese medicines do have a certain effect on the treatment of tumors; in particular, **studies on Fuzheng Peiben in the treatment of malignant tumors have shown that Fuzheng traditional Chinese medicine can enhance physical fitness, improve human immune function, improve quality of life and prolong survival.**

However, TCM treatment of tumors is mostly based on clinical experience observation, and no experimental research has been carried out.

In order to explore whether the spleen strengthening, qi nourishing and nourishing methods in the traditional Chinese medicine can effectively inhibit the growth of tumors, we conducted the following experiments.

2. The method

This experiment had the following groups:

Buzhong Yiqi (group A, n = 20),

Qi and blood supplement (group B, n=20),

Nourish kidney yin (group C, n=20),

Warming and nourishing kidney-yang (group D, n=20),

Combat and supplement ATCA mixture (group E, 11=20),

Xiao Chaihu Decoction (group F, n 2 20) and compound capsules (group G, n = 20), which were used to treat S180-bearing mice, systematically observed the appearance time, tumor growth, and survival time of each group of mice's tumors, their serum protein content, peripheral blood T lymphocyte count and immune organ weight were measured.

3. The results

The results showed as the followings:

Fuzheng Peiben and the ATCA mixture mainly composed of Fuzheng Peiben can significantly delay the appearance of tumors in vaccinated mice.

Inhibit tumor growth (the tumor inhibition rates in groups A, B, C, D, and E were 40%, 45%, 44.5%, 31% and 36%, respectively),

The extended survival time of tumor-bearing mice (the prolongation rates of survival in groups A, B, C, D, and E were 27.6, 45%, 38.5%, 25% and 26.5%, respectively).

Xiaochaihu Decoction and Compound Capsules, which mainly eliminate evils, cannot significantly inhibit tumor growth and prolong survival (compared with E group, P>0.05).

<u>**The levels of serum proteins in groups A, B, C, D, and E increased, the ratio of A/G increased, and the count of peripheral blood T lymphocytes increased**</u>

(compared with group G, P<0.05, group B, C, P<0.01), Thymus atrophy is obviously suppressed.

In conclusion:

This study shows that Fuzheng Peiben or the treatment based on Fuzheng Peiben is more effective in suppressing tumors and enhancing immunity than the treatment based on eliminating pathogens.

This experiment also observed the pregnancy of 7 tumor-bearing mice, of which 3 cases of pregnancy and postpartum tumor growth accelerated, **4 cases of tumor disappeared**.

It shows that pregnancy may have two different effects on tumor growth, and further observation and research are needed. It shows that pregnancy may have two different effects on tumor growth, and further observation and research are needed.

The first part

The experimental Observation of Fuzheng Peiben on Tumor Inhibition of S180-bearing Mice

Through more than 40 years of research and practice in the prevention and treatment of malignant tumors with integrated Chinese and Western medicine in my country, it has been found that many Chinese medicines do have a certain effect on the treatment of tumors. In particular, studies on Fuzheng Peiben in the treatment of malignant tumors show that Fuzheng traditional Chinese medicine can enhance physical fitness, improve human immunity, improve quality of life and prolong survival.

However, TCM treatment of tumors is mostly based on clinical experience observation, and no experimental research has been carried out.

In order to investigate whether the spleen, qi, blood and kidney-tonifying drugs in the Chinese and Western Strengthening and Strengthening Pei Ben can effectively inhibit tumor growth, the following experimental study was designed.

1. Materials and methods

1). Experimental animal

160 Kunming mice, 5-6 weeks old, weighing 27±2g, half male and half (provided by the Animal Center of Hubei Academy of Medical Sciences).

2). **Tumor-bearing animal model**

The SI80 ascites tumor strain was provided by Hubei Provincial Tumor Hospital. 1X107X0.2ml tumor cell suspension was respectively inoculated into each experimental mouse's right forelimb axilla subcutaneously.

3). **The Experiment grouping**

The experimental animals were randomly divided into:

Group A: Buzhong Yiqi treatment group (n=20);
Group B: Qi and blood double tonic treatment group (n=20);
Group C: Nourishing Kidney Yin Treatment Group (n=20);
Group D: Warming and nourishing kidney-yang treatment group (n=20);
Group E: ATCA mixture treatment group (n=20);
Group F: Xiaochaihu Decoction treatment group (n=20);
Group G: Compound xx capsule treatment group (n=20);
Group H: tumor-bearing control group (n=20).

Starting from the second day after vaccination, each group was given 0.4ml of traditional Chinese medicine per day.

The tumor-bearing control group was treated with the same amount of normal saline.

4). **The preparation of Chinese medicines in each group**

(1) Replenishing the middle energy and qi:

The main ingredients are xx, xx, etc. According to the original formula of Li Dongyuan's "Spleen and Stomach Theory", it is converted into a modern dosage and made by decoction, and the concentration of crude drug is 200%.

(2) Double nourishment of qi and blood:

The main ingredients are xx, xx, xx, etc. According to the original formula of "Medical Invention", it is made by decoction and concentration, and the concentration of crude drug is 200%.

(3) Nourish kidney yin:

The main ingredients are xx, xx, xx, etc. According to Qian Yi's "Pediatric Medicine Syndrome Direct Jue", the original formula is converted into a modern dose and it is made by decoction and concentration, with a crude drug concentration of 200%.

(4) Warming kidney and strengthening yang:

The main ingredients are xx, xx, xx, etc. According to Zhang Ji's "Golden Plaque Synopsis", the original formula is converted into a modern dosage and it is made by decoction, and the concentration of crude drug is 200%.

(5) Combination of attack and supplement (ATCA mixture): The main ingredients are xx, xx, etc.

(6) Xiao Chai Hu Tang:

The main ingredients are xx, xx, xx, etc. According to Zhang Ji's "Treatise on Febrile Diseases", the original formula is converted into a modern dosage and it is decocted and concentrated. The concentration of crude drug is 200%.

(7) Compound Tianx Capsule No. 1:

The main ingredients are xx, xx, etc. 0.5g/capsule, 60 capsules/bottle. Dissolve in distilled water to make a 3% Tianx capsule solution.

The above drug concentration is obtained after the normal human dose is converted to the mouse dose, and the conversion formula is as follows:

$$D2 = D1 \times R2 \times R1$$

Where:

D2-Mice dosage;

D1-human dose;

R1-R value of human body;

R2:-The corresponding R value for mice

5). *Observation item*

(1) Observation of tumor growth:

After inoculation with tumor cells, observe the appearance time of tumor nodules (days), measure the weight (g) of each mouse every 3 days, and measure the size of tumor nodules (maximum diameter mm X vertical transverse diameter mm) with a vernier caliper.

(2) Comparison of tumor suppression at all levels:

For all experimental mice that died or were put to death, the tumor tissue was completely removed after weighing, and the tumor tissue weight was weighed with a balance to calculate the tumor inhibition rate of each treatment group. The formula is as follows:

Control group tumor weight/weight-treatment group tumor weight/weight

Tumor inhibition rate = _____ X100%

Control group tumor weight/body weight

(3) Survival observation of each group:

Observe the hair, quality of life and survival period (days) of mice in each group. Calculate the survival rate of each group, the formula is as follows:

Average survival of the treatment group-average survival of the control group

Longer survival rate= x _____ 100%

Mean survival time of control group

(4) Determination of serum albumin and total protein:

The albumin was measured by the cresol green method, and the total protein was measured by the double-shrinking pulse method.

The kits are all produced by Beijing Chemical Plant.

In each group, 5 mice were sacrificed in the 2nd and 4th weeks after inoculation, their albumin and total protein content were measured, and the corresponding globulin content and the ratio of albumin (A)/globulin (C) were calculated.

(5) Dynamic observation of T lymphocyte count in peripheral blood:

Peripheral blood T lymphocytes were counted using a-acetate lipase staining method, 200 lymphocytes were counted, and the percentage of T lymphocytes was calculated.

(6) Weight measurement of thymus and spleen:

The experimental mice were sacrificed, dissected, the thymus and spleen were completely removed, their size was observed, and weighed with a torsion balance, and the thymus and wet weight of the spleen (mg)/body weight (g) of each mouse were calculated.

2. The Experimental results

1. Comparison of tumor appearance time in each group

See Table 1.

Table 1
Comparison of tumor appearance time in each group

Group	N	Tumor appearance time (d) (X±SD)	Earliest time (day)	Latest appearance time {day}
A	10	9.4±3.6*	5	15
B	10	12.5±5.3**	5	None
C	10	10.7±4.5*	4	21
D	10	9.7± 4.0*	4	15
E	10	10.9±5.4*	4	None
F	10	5.6 ± 4.9	4	6
G	10	6.3 ± 4.5	4	15
H	10	6.0		

Note: In the table *Compared with H group, P<0.05; **Compared with H group, P<0.01

It can be seen from Table 1 that the appearance time of tumors in the tumor-bearing control group was 6.0 days, and the tumor appearance times in the A, B, C, D, and E groups were 9.4, 12.5, 10.7, 9.7, and 10.9 days, respectively, which were similar to those in the tumor-bearing control group, was significant differences from the control group.

It shows that the medicine of Fuzheng Pei has the effect of delaying the appearance of tumor, that is, replenishing qi and blood.

Nourishing yin and tonifying the kidney, etc. can significantly prolong the appearance time of tumor inoculation. The earliest tumor appearance time of each treatment group is roughly the same, but the latest tumor appearance time varies greatly between groups, with the largest difference being 21 days. Individual experimental mice never showed tumors. It may be related to medication and pregnancy (below), or to improper operation of tumor inoculation. Because S180 tumor cell suspension is easy to precipitate under static state, it must be shaken every time it is used.

It can also be seen from Table 1 that Xiaochaihu Decoction and Compound Tianx Capsules have no significant effect on the appearance time of tumors, that is, treatments such as heat-clearing and detoxification cannot prolong the appearance time of inoculated tumors.

2. The observation of tumor nodule size in each group of mice

In this experiment, a quasi-clinical method was used to establish medical records for each mouse, and the tumor nodules (maximum diameter x vertical transverse diameter) mm2 were measured with a cursor card every 2 days, and the geometric mean was taken as the average vertical diameter of the mouse tumor. The final measured value of all death cases will be used as the subsequent measurements in the same group.

3. The comparison of tumor inhibition rate in each group

See Table 2. In each group, 5 experimental mice were killed at the 2nd and 4th week respectively to compare the tumor inhibition rate of each group. It can be seen from Table 6-2 that at the 2nd week, the tumor weight (g)/body weight (g) of groups B and C Compared with the tumor-bearing control group, there are significant differences, while the other treatment groups have no significant differences compared with the tumor-bearing control group.

At the 4ᵗʰ week of treatment, the A, B, C, D, and E groups were significantly different from the tumor-bearing control group. The above shows that as the treatment progresses, the anti-tumor effect of the Fuzheng Peiben drug treatment group is increasing Obviously, but the F and G groups did not significantly inhibit S180. In this experiment, it was also observed that the number of tumor metastases in each Fuzheng Peiben drug treatment group was less than that of the control group.

Table 2

The comparison of tumor inhibition rate in each group

Unit: g

Group	N	Week 2		Week 4	
		Tumor weight/ weight X±SD	Tumor inhibition rate (%)	Tumor weight/ weight X±SD	Tumor inhibition rate (%)
A	10	0.039±0.011	11	0.095±0.015	40
B	10	0.024±0.008*	45.5	0. 087 ± 0. 028 *	45
C	10	0.023 ± 0.009 *	47.7	0.088±0.026*	44.5
D	10	0.036 ± 0.014	18.2	0.110±0.025 *	31
E	10	0.033±0.010	2.3	0.101 ± 0.039*	36
F	10	0.055 ± 0.012	- 25	0.166±0.081	-4.4
G	10	0.048±0.024	-10	0.149±0.060	6
H	10	0.044±0.014		0.159±0.040	

Note: Compared with group H, $P<0.05$

4. The comparison of the survival time of mice in each group

It can be seen from Table 6-3 that there is no significant difference in survival between the Xiaochaihu Decoction and Compound xx capsule treatment group and the tumor-bearing control group. The other treatment groups can significantly prolong the survival time of tumor-bearing mice. Among them, the qi and blood supplement treatment Compared with the tumor-bearing control group, there are very significant differences.

Each Fuzheng Peiben treatment group not only prolonged the survival period, but also had better hair and quality of life than the control group. Some experimental mice also had normal fertility and delivery capabilities.

Table 3
Comparison of the survival time of mice in each group

Group	N	Lifetime (d)	Survival extension rate (%)
A	10	45.7 ± 6.4*	27.6
B	10	52.2 ± 6.9 **	45.0
C	10	49.6 ± 7.2 *	38.5
D	10	44.7 ± 8.4*	25.0
E	10	45.3 ± 6.4*	26.5
F	10	36.2 ± 4.8	1.1
G	10	36.9 ± 7.6	2.8
H	10	35.8±8.6	

Note: ●Compared with H group, P<0. 05; ***Compared with H group, P<0. 01

5. The comparison of serum protein (A), globulin (G) and albumin/globulin ratio of each group

See Table 4.

Table 4

The comparison of albumin, globulin and white/ball ratio of each group

Group	N	Week 2			Week 4		
		A(g) X± SD	G(g)X±SD	A/G	A(g)X±SD	G(g)X±SD	A/G
A	10	1.54± 0.17*	3.44±0.21	0.45	1.46±0.18 *	3.40 ± 0.22	0.43
B	10	1.56±0.14*	3.42 ± 0.20	0.46	1.49 ± 0.15*	3.54 ± 0.23	0.42
C	10	1. 55 ± 0.13 *	3.46±0.21	0.45	1.45±0.13*	3.51±0.20	0.41
D	10	1.51±0.12 *	3.44 ± 0.23	0.44	1.47±0.15	3.46 ± 0.19	0.42
E	10	1.48±0.16*	3.31±0.19	0.45	1.38 ± 0.14 *	3.25±0.21	0.42
F	10	1.41± 0.27	3.48± 0.24	0.41	1.25±0.15	3.30± 0.22	0.37
G	10	1.38 ± 0.24	3.40 ± 0.20	0.45	1.24±0.16	3.29 ± 0.28	0.38
H	10	1.33±0.14	3. 33 ± 0.20	0.40	1.21±0.13	3.27±0.18	0.37

Note: *Compared with group H, $P<0.05$

In each group, 5 experimental mice were sacrificed at the 2nd and 4th weeks after treatment, the eyeballs were taken to take blood, and the serum albumin and globulin contents were measured. It can be seen from Table 4 that at the 2nd week, A, B, The albumin content of, C, D, E groups was significantly different from that of the tumor-bearing control group. There was no significant difference in globulin between the groups, and the A/C ratio of each treatment group was higher than that of the tumor-bearing control group. At the 4th week, the albumin and globulin values of each group decreased, and the A/C ratio decreased, but the albumin content of groups A, B, C, D, and E was still significantly different from that of group H.

The above shows that as the tumor progresses, the serum protein of tumor-bearing mice decreases progressively. This is consistent with the decrease of protein content in clinical tumor patients, and the appearance of weight loss, late stage cachexia, and systemic failure. The application of Fuzheng Pei medicine can increase the serum whiteness of tumor-bearing mice. Protein content, increase the A/C ratio.

6. The dynamic observation of T lymphocyte count in peripheral blood

It can be seen from Table 6-5 that the T lymphocytes of the tumor-bearing control group are significantly lower than those of the normal control group (the T lymphocyte count of the normal control group X=61.5±2.0, N=10), indicating that the development of tumors has an effect on cellular immunity The inhibition of function is positive. As the tumor progressed, T lymphocytes in the tumor-bearing control group further decreased. The I lymphocyte count of each treatment group was significantly different from the control group at the first week, second week, and fourth week, except for the F and C groups. By the 6th week, the T lymphocytes of each treatment group decreased, and there was no significant difference from the tumor-bearing control group. Combined with the tumor growth, in the first week, second week, and fourth week, although the tumor growth in each righting treatment group, the drug began to exert tumor suppression effect, and the level of T lymphocytes increased; but by the sixth week, the tumor in each treatment group had already Increase, the level of T lymphocytes also further decline.

7. The measurement of wet weight of thymus and spleen in each group

Table 5

Dynamic observation of T lymphocyte count in peripheral blood

Group	N		T lymphocyte count (%) X ± SD								
		n	1W	n	2W	n	4W	n	6W
A	10	10	37.3 ± 6.8*	10	36.4 ± 5.5*	9	41.5 ± 4.2*	4	35.2±4.4
B	10	10	39.8 ± 10.6 *	10	41.5 ± 3.8* *	9	44.8 ± 3.8* *	7	41.2 ± 3.5
C	10	10	37.8 ± 6.3*	10	43.2 ± 3.4* *	10	38.6 ± 5.6* *	5	32.4±4.2
D	10	10	37.4± 5.8 *	10	39.6 ± 8.0*	8	37.5 ± 5.9*	4	31.5 ± 2.4
E	10	10	36.6± 4.9*	10	37.3 ± 4.8*	8	35.6 ± 4.2	5	
F	10	10	36.4 ± 6.3	10	34.0 ± 5.98	8	30.4 ± 2.1	0	-
G	10	10	34.1± 5.0	10	32.4 ± 3.1	6	29.5 ± 4.7	0	-
H	10	10	32.1 ± 3.6	10	30.1 ± 5.8	6	28.7 ± 6.8	1	39.5

Note: *Compared with group H, P<0.05

Part of the experimental mice were sacrificed in the 2nd and 4th weeks respectively, and the thymus and spleen were dissected and weighed. The thymus index and spleen index of each group were calculated and compared with the normal control group and the tumor-bearing control group (see Table 6).

Table 6

Thymus and spleen weight/weight comparison in each group

Group	N	Thymus (mg)/ body weight (g)	X ± SD	Spleen (mg)/ body weight (g)	X ± SD
		Week 2	Week 4	Week 2	Week 4
A	10	2.50 ± 0.34 *	0.40±0.50#	4.84±1.06	4. 20 ± 0.98
B	10	2. 58 ± 0.42 *	2.54±0.40#**	4.96±0.92	4. 22 ± 0.82
C	10	2.55±0.38 *	2.48 ± 0.33 *	4.82±0.48	4.16±0.58
D	10	2.48±0.33*	2.40±0.48#	* 4.95±0.65	4.24±0.88
E	10	2. 47 ± 0.28 *	2.44±0.39#	4.67±0.58	4.30 ± 0.69
F	10	1. 46± 0. 23##	1.24±0.41##	4.20±0.5	54.01±0.76
G	10	1.56±0.36#	1.24±0.39##	4.45±0.79	3.67±0.91
H	10	1. 72± 0. 30#	1.06±0.29##	4.20 ± 0.82	3.98± 0.80

Note: *Compared with H group, P<0.05; **Compared with H group, P<0.01;;#Compared with normal control group, P<0. 05;##Compared with normal control group, P<0.01

It can be seen from Table 6 that the thymus of the tumor-bearing control group was significantly atrophied compared with the normal group (P <0.05) (the thymus of the normal control group/body weight (mg/g)X=2.90±0.40, n=10), with Tumor progression, Thymu. The shrinkage became more pronounced. In the second week of the tumor course, all treatment groups except F and G groups were significantly different from the tumor-bearing control group, indicating that Fuzheng Peiben Chinese medicine has a certain effect on inhibiting the atrophy of tumor-bearing mice Thymus; at the fourth week, each treatment Thymus in the group were atrophied, but there was still a significant difference from the tumor-bearing control group, and also significantly different from the normal control group. The anatomy showed that the thymus glands of each group of tumor-bearing mice were atrophied. The diameter of the thymus glands decreased from 5-7mm in the normal range to 2-4mm in the second week and 1-12mm in the fourth week. The thymus glands were dark in color and brittle in texture. Combined with the tumor growth, the tumor was smaller in the second week, and the thymus index of each treatment group had decreased; the tumor was larger in the fourth week, and the thymus/body weight was even lower. Observation of the thymus and body weight of each group of tumor-bearing mice showed that the larger the tumor, the smaller the thymus; the smaller the tumor, the larger the thymus, and the two were negatively correlated. The changes in the spleen were not as obvious as those in the thymus. The spleens of each experimental mouse were congested and swollen, increased in volume, increased in weight, dark red in color, and brittle in texture. In the late stage of the tumor, the spleen was relatively atrophy, and there was no significant difference between the treatment groups and the normal control group and the tumor-bearing control group.

3. Discussion

1). *The effect of Fuzheng Peiben therapy on tumor suppression and survival*

In clinical practice, many tumor patients show symptoms of deficiency, such as deficiency of qi, deficiency of blood, deficiency of yin and deficiency of yang. Therefore, the treatment should be used to strengthen the body to strengthen the body. This experiment explored the methods of strengthening the body and strengthening the body and the anti-tumor effects of both attacking and supplementing. The results showed that: the strengthening of the body and the treatment of strengthening the body, such as nourishing the middle and nourishing qi, qi and blood, nourishing kidney yin and warming and invigorating the kidney yang, etc. The main ATCA mixture can significantly delay the time of tumor inoculation in mice, inhibit tumor growth, and prolong the survival time of tumor-bearing mice. Analyzed from the tumor inhibition rate of each group: in the qi and blood double supplement experimental group, its tumor inhibition rate reached 45%; in the nourishing kidney yin experimental group, its tumor inhibition rate reached 44.5%, followed by invigorating the middle and replenishing qi, and The anti-tumor effect is also

40%, and the effect is also good; again, the ATCA mixture, the tumor suppression rate is 36%; but the warming and nourishing kidney-yang treatment group has a poorer effect, with a tumor suppression rate of 31%; it seems that it should be used for tumor suppression Therapeutic method of nourishing qi and blood and nourishing kidney yin. Analyzed from the prolongation rate of survival: the qi and blood double supplement group reached 45%, which was the longest survival group; the second was the nourishing kidney-yin group, reaching 38.5%, and the effect was also good; as for invigorating the middle and replenishing qi, warming The ATCA mixture treatment group of nourishing kidney-yang and attacking and replenishing can also prolong survival, but it is not as good as the treatment group of nourishing qi and blood and nourishing kidney-yin. The Xiaochaihu Decoction and Compound Tianx Capsule treatment group, which mainly eliminates evils, showed in this group of experiments that it could not significantly inhibit the tumor, nor could it prolong the survival period of mouse tumors, and its effect was the worst. Therefore, from the aspect of prolonging survival, the treatment of qi and blood supplementing and nourishing kidney yin is the first choice, followed by supplementing the middle and replenishing qi, warming the kidney yang, and attacking and tonic. In terms of both inhibiting tumors and prolonging survival time, the best way to replenish qi and blood is to nourish the kidney yin, followed by a mixture of tonifying the middle and replenishing qi and ATCA. The therapeutic effect of warming and tonifying the kidney yang is not obvious. As for Xiaochaihu Decoction and Fufang Tianx Capsules, which mainly eliminate evil, there is no obvious effect from the results of this experiment. In a word, the treatments based on Fuzheng culture and the treatment based on Fuzheng culture have the effect of inhibiting tumor growth and prolonging survival to varying degrees, while the treatment based on eliminating pathogens has no obvious effect of inhibiting tumor and prolonging survival.

In other words: the treatment based on eliminating evil has no effect.

This experiment shows that Fuzheng Peiben or treatment based on Fuzheng Peiben has obvious anti-tumor effect on smaller tumors, and can significantly prolong survival and improve the quality of life. Therefore, it is mostly used clinically as postoperative radiotherapy and chemotherapy. One of the auxiliary treatment methods. Many literature reports that the clinical use of Fuzheng Peiben to treat malignant tumors has achieved good results. The results of this experiment further confirm that therapies such as dual qi and blood, nourishing kidney yin, and nourishing middle and nourishing qi can inhibit tumors and prolong survival. The combination of western medicine and clinical treatment of malignant tumors provides experimental evidence.

2). *The effect of Fuzheng Peiben therapy on enhancing the body's immunity*

This experiment shows that both Fuzheng Peiben and Fuzheng Peiben-based treatments can increase the level of peripheral blood T lymphocytes to varying degrees. For example, at the 4th week, the T lymphocyte levels are as follows: Buzhong Yiqi group 41.5%, 44.8% in the qi and blood supplementing group, 38.6% in the nourishing kidney-yin group, 37.5% in the warming and invigorating kidney-yang group, and 35.6 in the ATCA mixture group; inhibiting thymic atrophy, such as in the second week, invigorating qi and qi and blood There were significant differences in the thymus index between the nourishing and nourishing kidney yin, warming the kidney and strengthening yang, and the thymus index of the ATCA mixture treatment group and the tumor-bearing control group. It is suggested that the anti-tumor effect of Fuzheng Peiben may be related to enhancing the body's immune function. Some people think that many plant polysaccharides have immunomodulators (immunenocclulator) properties, called anti-tumor polysaccharides. These polysaccharides cannot directly kill cancer cells, but they can activate the body's immune system to release cytokines with anti-tumor effects or enhance LAK cell response. The killing effect of cancer cells. Fuzheng Pei is rich in plant polysaccharides. As reported by Zhao Kesheng, Huangmao polysaccharides were extracted and found to have a molecular weight of 20 000 to 25,000 components, which can secrete tumor necrosis in vitro on peripheral blood mononuclear cells (PBMC) of normal people and tumor patients. Factor (TNF) has a significant promoting effect. Chen Kai et al. reported: Chinese medicine compound Fuzheng Anticancer Liquid on transplanted tumor S18. Mouse natural killer cell activity and interleukin 2 (IL-2) activity have a promoting effect, and can promote the remnant of T lymphocytes, promote the phagocytic function of peritoneal macrophages, and increase the weight of spleen and thymus. In short, the effect of Fuzheng Peiben on the human immune system is very complicated and needs further observation and research.

3). *Fuzheng Peiben treatment enhances the human body's ability to fight disease, enhances blood cells and enhances physical strength. This experiment shows that*:

Strengthening the vitality and training instinct can increase the serum protein content of tumor-bearing mice and increase the white/globulin ratio. Studies have shown that: postoperative application of esophageal cancer, gastric cancer, colorectal cancer + Fuzheng Pei this medicine. RBC. Hb were higher than the control group, and the reduction of white blood cells was also suppressed. It shows that the instinct of strengthening the body can improve blood cells and protein, strengthen physical strength, and improve disease resistance. Fuzheng Peiben has been widely used clinically as one of the treatments of integrated traditional Chinese and Western medicine for the treatment of tumors. The results of this experiment show that Fuzheng Peiben therapy can delay the appearance of tumors in inoculated mice, inhibit tumor growth, prolong the survival time of tumor-bearing mice, enhance the body's immune function and disease resistance, and improve the quality of life. It can provide experimental basis for clinical Chinese medicine anti-cancer.

The second part

The experimental observation on the effect of pregnancy on tumor growth in S180-bearing mice

In order to explore the effect of pregnancy on tumor growth in S180-bearing mice, the following experimental studies were designed.

1. Materials and methods

1) The experimental animals are the same as Experiment 1.

2) Tumor-bearing animal model

3) The experiment grouping

4) The observation index is as the followings:

① Observe the number of days from inoculation to conception of each mouse, changes in tumor nodule size during conception and delivery, postpartum tumor growth and postpartum survival (days);

② Count of T lymphocytes in peripheral blood of each pregnant mouse:

The counting method of peripheral blood T lymphocytes is the same as experiment 1. Observe the T lymphocyte counts of each mouse before conception, during pregnancy and 1 week after delivery.

2. The experimental results

1). *Changes of tumor size and postpartum survival period of each mouse before and after pregnancy vibration*

From Table 7, it can be seen that 2 cases of mice in group B became pregnant, of which 1 case of postpartum tumor growth accelerated and died within 14 days; 1 case of postpartum tumor disappeared and lasted for 4 weeks; 2 cases of group C became pregnant and both were receiving tumors On the second day after the cell, 1 case of tumor appeared and disappeared after delivery for 4 weeks; 1 case never appeared tumor; 3 cases in group H were pregnant, 1 case had tumor at conception, and the tumor disappeared during delivery for 4 weeks; 2 cases There was no tumor at conception, but the tumor continued to grow after delivery during pregnancy, and died on 22 and 5 days after delivery, respectively. It shows that pregnancy, breastfeeding and the application of drugs may affect growth. Because the number of observation cases is too small, it is difficult to summarize the rules, and further experimental observation is needed.

Table 7

The comparison of tumor size before and after pregnancy
and postpartum survival time of each mouse

Group	Rat	Vaccination to pregnant (d)	Tumor size before and after pregnancy (mm)		Postpartum tumor	Postpartum survival period (d)
			pregnant period	delivery time		
B	8	30	6x5	22x15	faster	14
B	9	24	3x3	no	disappearance lasts 4 weeks	long-term survival
C	7	1	no	5x5	disappears for 4 weeks	long-term survival
C	10	1	no	no	no	long-term survival
H	1	7	3x4	No	no	long-term survival
H	6	7	without	11x 11	faster	22
H	7	12	no	11x8	faster	5

Note: Long-term survival means the survival period exceeds 3 months

2). *The dynamic Observation of T Lymphocytes in Peripheral Blood Before and After Pregnant Women*

It can be seen from Table 6-8 that the counts of T lymphocytes in each mouse increased during pregnancy, and those with T lymphocytes tended to decline one week after delivery, the tumor grew faster, and the prognosis was poor; for those with increased T lymphocytes after delivery, all tumors disappeared and the rat can be the long-term survival.

It shows that T lymphocyte count is one of the useful indicators for judging the prognosis of pregnant tumor-bearing mice.

Table 8

Peripheral blood T lymphocyte count of each pregnant mouse

Group	Rat	T lymphocyte count		
		Before conception	Pregnancy period	1 week after delivery
B	8	31.5	34	28
B	9	39	48	55
C	7	-	42	53
C	10	-	47	58
H	1	33.5	37.5	39
H	6	35	36	30
H	7	35	36	-

3. Discussion

1). The effect of pregnancy vibration on tumor growth

It can be seen from the above data that pregnancy has a great influence on tumor growth: on the one hand, it may accelerate tumor growth, on the other hand, it may inhibit tumor growth. There are 160 tumor-bearing mice in this experimental group, of which 7 were pregnant.

Among these 7 pregnant mice, 3 cases died due to the acceleration of tumor growth postpartum, and 4 cases of postpartum tumor disappeared without recurring.

2). The effect of estrogen and progesterone on tumor growth

(1) Aspects that promote tumor growth:

Tan Duanjun reported that physiological concentration of estradiol has a certain growth stimulating effect on SGC-7901 cells, and benzoxamine can partially inhibit this effect. Feng Youji used proliferating cell nuclear antigen immunohistochemical method and nuclear division count to detect human ovarian epithelial (cell) carcinoma AO cells after co-cultured with FSH and LH for 48 hours. The results showed that FSH and LH promote ovarian epithelial cancer AO cells proliferation. The above shows that estrogen can promote tumor growth.

(2) Inhibition of tumor growth:

Song Liangnian et al. believe that cancer cells are undifferentiated and over-proliferating cells. Under the action of differentiation inducers, certain cancer cells can return to the normal differentiation track.

Someone used immunohistochemistry and flow cytometry to detect the expression of oncogene C-erbB2 in human epithelial ovarian cancer 3A0 cells co-cultured with medroxyprogesterone for 3 days. The results suggest: the anti-cancer effect of progesterone and cancer suppression Gene expression, which leads to a decrease in the carcinogenicity of cells, has also been reported. Peripheral blood mononuclear cells (PBMC) cultured in vitro can be stimulated by estradiol to produce TNF.

The above shows that progesterone can induce and suppress the expression of oncogenes through differentiation, or produce anti-cancer effects by activating immune factors. In short, the effect of estrogen and progesterone on tumor growth is very complicated, but it is not yet fully understood and needs further study.

2

The experimental research and clinical verification work that has been carried out

(1) The experimental research work

Our laboratory has carried out the following experimental studies to screen new anti-cancer and anti-metastatic drugs from Chinese medicine:

1). In vitro screening test:

Use cancer cell culture in vitro to observe the direct damage of cancer cell drugs to cancer cells. Put crude drug crude powder products (500ug/ml) into the test tubes for culturing cancer cells to observe whether they have an inhibitory effect on cancer cells and their tumor inhibition rate.

2). In vivo tumor suppression screening test:

Manufacture of cancer-bearing animal models, and conduct experimental screening studies on the anti-tumor rate of Chinese herbal medicines in cancer-bearing animals:

In each batch of experiments, 240 mice were divided into 8 experimental groups, each with 30 mice. The seventh group was the blank control group, and the eighth group used 5-Fu or CTX as the control group.

The whole group of mice were inoculated with EAC or S180 or H22 cancer cells. After 24 hours of inoculation, each mouse was orally fed with crude and raw rug powder and fed with the selected traditional Chinese medicine for a long time. The survival period was observed and the tumor inhibition rate was calculated.

In this way, we conducted experimental studies for 4 consecutive years, using more than 1,000 tumor-bearing animal models each year; in 4 years, we made nearly 6,000 tumor-bearing animal models. After each experimental mouse died, the liver, spleen, lung, and thymus were performed. Pathological anatomy of the kidney, more than 20,000 sections were performed.

3). Experimental results:

Among the 200 Chinese herbal medicines screened by animal experiments in our laboratory, _48 kinds of Chinese herbal medicines were screened out to have certain or even excellent inhibitory effects on cancer cells, with a tumor suppression rate of over 75-90%._ In this group, 152 species were screened and eliminated by animal experiments without obvious anticancer effects.

(2) Clinical verification

Based on the success of animal experiments, it was to carry out clinical verification:

1)). **Method:**

a. To establish an oncology specialist outpatient clinic and an anti-cancer, anti-metastasis, and recurrence research collaboration team with integrated Chinese and Western medicine;

b. To keep outpatient medical records;

c. To establish a complete follow-up observation system, and observe long-term effects.

d. It was from experimental research to clinical verification, when new problems are discovered in the clinical verification process, then it was to return to the laboratory for basic research, and then it was to apply the new experimental results to the clinic.

In this way, it was from the experiment to the clinical to the re-experiment to the re-clinical. All experimental research must pass clinical verification in a large number of patients for 3-5 years or even 8-10 years of observation,

According to evidence-based medicine, there are long-term follow-up and evaluable data.

<u>The efficacy criteria are:</u>
<u>Good quality of life and long life span and long survival term.</u>
<u>The result:</u>

<u>XZ-C immunomodulatory anti-cancer traditional Chinese medicine preparations have achieved remarkable results for the effects of cure and treatment or achieved significantly curative effects after they have been applied and observed by a large number of patients with advanced cancer.</u>

2)). Clinical data:

Anticancer Research Cooperation Group of combination of Chinese and Western Medicine and Shuguang Oncology Specialty Clinic used XZ-C immunomodulatory anticancer Chinese medicine to treat 4698 cases of stage III, IV or metastatic or recurring cancer, including 3051 males and 1647 females, the youngest 11 years old, up to 86 years old.

All patients in the group have been diagnosed by pathology or CT, MRI, B-ultrasound imaging. According to the International Anti-Cancer Alliance staging standards, all cases are stage III or higher in advanced patients, including:

1021 liver cancer cases, 752 cases of lung cancer, 694 cases of gastric cancer, 624 cases of esophagus and cardia cancer, 328 cases of rectal cancer, 442 cases of colon cancer, 368 cases of breast cancer, 74 cases of pancreatic cancer, 30 cases of cholangiocarcinoma, 43 cases of retroperitoneal tumor, 38 cases of ovarian cancer Cases, 9 cases of cervical cancer, 11 cases of brain tumor, 34 cases of thyroid cancer, 38 cases of nasopharyngeal cancer, 9 cases of melanoma, 27 cases of kidney cancer, 48 cases of bladder cancer, 13 cases of leukemia, 47 cases of supraclavicular metastasis, various kinds of sarcoma were 35 cases and 39 cases of other malignant tumors, etc.

3)). Drugs and methods of administration:

<u>The rule for treatment is to protect Thymus and to promote immune function and to protect bone marrow hematopoietic function, thereby enhancing the host's immune surveillance and controlling the immune escape of cancer cells.</u>

<u>From the perspective of traditional Chinese medicine, the treatment principle is to strengthen the body and eliminate the evil, soften the firmness and dispel the knots, and tonic both the qi and blood.</u>

The drugs are XZ-C1, XZ-C2, XZ-C3, XZ-C4, XZ-C5, XZ-C6, XZ-C7, XZ-C8... XZ-C10.

Depending on the different cancers, the disease conditions, and the metastasis situations, according to the dialectic of the disease condition it is to choose the above drugs.

Solid tumors or metastatic tumors were treated by both oral anti-cancer powder and external anti-tumor detumescence ointment. The external anti-cancer analgesic ointment for those with pain.

Patients with jaundice and ascites should use Tuihuang Decoction or Xiaoshui Decoction.

4)). *Treatment results:*

The symptoms are improved, the quality of life is improved, and the survival period is prolonged.

(1) Among the 4277 patients with advanced cancer who took XZ-C1-10 immunomodulatory Chinese medicine for more than 3 months, the medical records have detailed observation records of the efficacy, see Table 1.

Table 1
Observation of curative effect of 4277 cases to comprehensively
improve the quality of life of patients with advanced cancer

Get better	Spirit	Appetite	Body Strengthen	General conditions improve	Weight gain	Sleep better	Improvement activities Ability activity Limited relief	Self-care Walking activity usual	Return to work Doing light work Change symptoms
Number of cases	4071	3986	2450	479	2938	1005	1038	3220	479
(%)	95.2	93 2	57.3	11. 2	68.7	23.5	24.3	75.3	11.2

All patients in this group are in the middle and advanced stage, and all have different degrees of symptom improvement after taking the medicine, with an effective rate of 93.2%.

In terms of improving the quality of life (according to the Karnofsky scoring standard), the average score is 50 before medication, and the average is increased to 80 after medication. The patients in this group have metastasis and dysfunction of different tissues and organs above stage III. In the past statistics of such patients it was reported that the median survival time is about 6 months.

The longest cases in this group have reached 18 years, and the average survival time of the remaining cases is more than 1 year.

One case of primary liver cancer in the left lobe of the liver, recurred in the right liver after resection, and has been treated with XZ-C alone for 18 years;

Another case of liver cancer has been taking XZ-C for 10 and a half years;

In 2 cases of liver cancer, there were multiple tumors in the liver. After taking XZ-C for half a year, the tumors completely disappeared after 2 CT re-examinations, and they have been stable for half a year.

One case of double kidney cancer had extensive metastasis to the abdominal cavity after one side was resected. After taking XZ-C medicine, he has completely returned to work.

3 cases of lung cancer could be removed by opening the chest for exploration. Long-term use of XZ-C has been 3 and a half years.

Two cases of remnant gastric cancer have been taking XZ-C medicine for 8 years.

3 cases of rectal cancer recurrence took XZ-C medicine for 3 years.

One case of breast cancer with metastasis to the liver and ribs has been taking medicine for 8 years.

A female patient with a walnut-sized lymph node mass in both groin and neck was diagnosed as non-Hodgkin's lymphoma by pathology. She could not receive chemotherapy due to financial difficulties. She had taken XZ-C1+XZ-C4+XZ-C2 for a long time. For 4 years, it is to have the monthly follow-up visits to the outpatient clinic to get medicine. It is generally in good condition.

One case of recurrence of bladder cancer after renal cancer surgery has 9 and a half years after taking XZ-C.

<u>The above cases are all patients in the middle and late stages who cannot undergo surgery, radiotherapy or chemotherapy. They are only treated with XZ-C drugs without other drugs.</u>

<u>So far, it still comes to the clinic every month for review and medicine.</u>

<u>After taking the medicine for a long time, the condition is controlled in a stable state, so that the body and the tumor are in a balanced state for a long time, and a better survival with the tumor is obtained, the patient's symptoms are improved, the quality of life is improved, and the survival period is prolonged.</u>

(2) For 84 patients with solid tumors and 56 patients with metastatic supraclavicular lymphadenopathy, after oral administration of XZ-C series and external or topical application of ointment of XZ-C3 anti-cancer softening firmness and dispelling hard mass, the good results have been obtained, as shown in Table 2.

Table 2

Changes of 84 cases of solid tumors and 56 cases of metastatic nodules after external application of XZ-C ointment

	Solid tumor mass				Swollen supraclavicular lymph nodes in the neck			
	Disappear	Reduced ½	Turn soft	No change	Disappear	Reduced ½	Turn soft	No change
Number of cases (%)	12 14.2	28 33.3	32 38.0	12 14.2	12 21.4	22 39.2	14 25.0	8 14.2
Total effective rate (%)				85.7				85.7

(3) 298 patients with cancer pain achieved significant pain relief effects by taking XZ-C medicine internally and applying XZ-C anticancer pain relief cream externally. See Table 3.

Table 3

Pain relief after oral administration of XZ-C drug and external
application of XZ-C anticancer pain relief ointment in 298 patients

Clinical manifestations	Pain			
	Mild relief	Significantly reduced	Disappear	Invalid
Number of cases	52	139	93	14
(%)	17.3	46.8	31.2	4.7
Total effective rate (%)		95.3		

3

The immunopharmacology of XZ-C immune regulation and control Chinese medications:

Compared with western medicine immunopharmacology, Chinese medicine immunopharmacology has its own characteristics and advantages. After long-term clinical experience, Chinese medicine has accumulated a large number of prescriptions to regulate the body's immune function, especially tonic Chinese medicines which generally have the benefit of regulating immune vitality.

Traditional Chinese medicines, whether single-medicine or prescriptions, will have multiple active ingredients, unlike western medicines (synthetic medicines) that have a single structure. The role of traditional Chinese medicine is multifaceted. *In addition to regulating immune function, it also has a certain effect on the overall function of each functional system.*

The main role of XZ-C Chinese medicine immunomodulators is to regulate cellular immunity and regulate immune response medicated by various immune cell (various immune cell-mediated immune responses), including cytokines or lymphokines.

The immunomodulatory function of traditional Chinese medicine mainly acts on stem cell immunity, such as on the thymus, gonads and lymphatic system, T, B cells and various cytokines.

Ancient Chinese medicine has the notion that righteous qi is not weak and evil qi is not invaded, which constitutes an integral part of traditional Chinese medicine theory. The essence is to maintain the overall functional balance and enhance disease resistance. Its main function is to enhance the body's immune function. In fact, tonic drugs are based on immunopharmacology.

Immunopharmacology is an emerging edge subject, which serves as a bridge between pharmacology and immunology.

The traditional Chinese medicine in XZ-C immunomodulator has obvious immune-promoting effect. It is an effective immune-promoting agent. This field is worthy of vigorous development. It should be explored to become a new type of immune-promoting agent, which it make it a reliable, effective and safe medicine for treating patients.

The Chinese herbal medicines (almost all tastes) in XZ-C4 basically, have the effect of immune booster. It has been proved in animal experiments to significantly promote the function of thymus.

<u>The main role of traditional Chinese medicine immunomodulators is to regulate cellular immunity and regulate immune responses mediated by various immune cells, including cytokines or lymphokines</u>.

4

Pharmacodynamics Study of XZ-C Immune regulation and control Chinese Medications

1). **Based on the above anti-cancer pharmacology and animal experiments, XZ-C drug has obvious anti-tumor effect.**

Tumor inhibitory effect of XZ-C Chinese medicine on H22 mice bearing liver cancer:

XZ-C1 tumor inhibition rate (the tumor inhibition rate of XZ-C1) at the 6th week was 58%;

XZ-C4 tumor inhibition rate at the 6th week is 70%;

The tumor inhibition rate of cyclophosphamide (CTX) at the 6th week was 49%.

The life extension rate of XZ-C1 is 98%, indicating that XZ-C drugs have good anti-cancer effects.

2). **XZ-C drug can increase efficacy and reduce toxicity of chemotherapy drugs.**

The 3rd and 6th anti-cancer pharmacology above-mentioned have shown that XZ-C4 has a better effect of increasing efficiency and reduced toxicity of anti-cancer drugs.

3). **XZ-C immune regulation and control anti-cancer Chinese medicine has the effect of protecting the function of hematopoietic system.**

Using MMC or Cyclophosphamide (CTX) in cancer-bearing mice caused chemotherapeutic drugs to inhibit the bone marrow hematopoietic system in WBC↓, PLT↓. After taking XZ-C4 for 4 weeks, Hb, WBC, and PLT were all significantly improved.

4). **XZ-C immune regulation and control anti-cancer Chinese medicine can protect immune organs and improve the immune function of the human body.**

After the above H22 cancer-bearing mice were treated with Cyclophosporine (CTX), the white blood cells decreased (there is leucopenia), the immune function was lowered (reduced immune function), and the kidney section was damaged(damage to kidney slices).

After the use of XZ-C4, the immune function can be significantly improved, and the white blood cells and the red blood cells can be increased. In the XZ-C treatment group, the thymus did not shrink and was slightly enlarged or hypertrophy, with dense lymphocytes and increased epithelial reticulocytes, or inside Thymus, lymphocytes are dense, and epithelial reticulocytes increase.

5

The research of XZ-C4 anti-cancer traditional Chinese medicine induces cytokine

(1) XZ-C4 can induce endogenous cytokines

1). After experimental research, XZ-C4 has a variety of immune enhancement effects, and it is closely related to the induction of endogenous cytokines.

2). XZ-C4 can inhibit the reduction of white blood cells, granulocytes and thrombocytopenia.

3). XZ-C4 not only has a direct effect on the production of granulocyte macrophage colony stimulating factor (GM-CSF) through interleukin-1ß (lL-1ß), but also can enhance tumor necrosis factor (TNF) and interferon (IFN) and other cytokines, the latter may be an indirect mechanism of action.

4). In cancer patients, Th1 cytokine, which regulates cellular immune function, has decreased, while XZ-C4 can increase it.

It is effective for anemia and leukopenia after chemotherapy.

5). Experimental analysis found that XZ-C4 not only protects the bone marrow, but also has a direct effect on the differentiation of cancer cells through cytokines.

In short, XZ-C4 exhibits various cytokines due to autocrine, which induces cell differentiation and natural death.

In short, XZ-C4 exhibits various cytokines due to autocrine, which induces cell differentiation and natural death.

The so-called autocrine refers to the substances secreted by oneself and in turn act on oneself.

Looking to the future, XZ-C4 may become an induction therapy for cancer cell differentiation.

(2) XZ-C4 can inhibit cancer progression and metastasis

Cancer cells acquire the malignant nature of infiltration and metastasis in the process of proliferation. Or in the process of proliferation, cancer cells acquire the malignant nature of infiltration and metastasis. This phenomenon is called the progression of malignancy, or this phenomenon is called malignant progression.

Research on cancer progression requires animal models with good reproducibility. Therefore, the regressive cancer cell QR-32 isolated from mouse fibrosarcoma was made into this reproducible model.

Even if QR-32 is implanted subcutaneously in mice, it will not proliferate, but will completely disappear on its own; if it is injected into a vein, there will be no metastatic nodules in the lung.

However, if gelatin sponge, which is a foreign body in the body, and QR-32 are implanted under the skin of mice, QR-32 will become proliferative cancer cell QR5P0 in vivo.

If QR5P is cultured in vitro and then transplanted into another mouse, tumors will grow even if there is no foreign body. If it is administered intravenously, lung metastasis will occur.

Using this model, we have completed research on whether XZ-C4 can affect cancer progression.

The progress of this model is divided into two processes:

That is, the process of OR-32 transforming into proliferative cancer cell CRSP (pre-stage progression) and the process of OR5 P proliferation into carcinoma (late stage progression).

After feeding with XZ-C4, the disease progression of the two types of model mice was inhibited, especially the most significant inhibition of the previous progress, and it was dependent on the dosage.

In terms of prolonging the survival time of model mice, all models transplanted with QR-32 and gelatin sponge at the same time died within 65 days, while 30% of mice with XZ-C4 survived 150 days after tumor transplantation.

Previous experiments and clinical studies believe that XZ-C4 can enhance the immune effect and reduce the side effects of cancer drugs.

This experimental study proved that XZ-C4 has the effect of inhibiting cancer progression. It can inhibit its infiltration and metastasis. Or this experimental study proved that XZ-C4 has the effect of inhibiting the progression of cancer, and can inhibit its invasion and metastasis.

6

The study on the Toxicology of XZ-C Immunomodulation Anti-cancer Traditional Chinese Medication

XZ-C1 can be taken for a long time.

The acute toxicity test shows:

The mice were intragastrically administered 100 times of the adult dose (10g/kg body weight). Observed at 24, 48, 72, and 96 hours respectively, none of the 30 purebred mice died.

LD50 is difficult to check out or to make and it is a fairly safe prescription.

According to the WHO "Acute and Acute Toxicity Classification Standards of Anticancer Drugs", it was to measure or to assess **the changes in peripheral blood, liver and kidney functions of patients after different doses and different dosage forms in order to understand their toxicity and side effects.**

More than 6000 cases of XZ-C drugs were taken orally, and the drugs were taken continuously for only 3 months, and some cases were as long as several years.

In these groups there were a small number of patients who had no abnormal change in WBC, RBC, Hb, and PLT while their blood tests were checked up before and after treatment; most of them had improved blood conditions, and Hb%, RBC, WBC, and PLT all increased.

In order to control tumors, many patients in our specialist clinics have taken XZ-C1+4 for a long time for 3-5 years.

Adhering to long-term medication can often stabilize the condition, inhibit the proliferation of cancer cells, improve the quality of life, and prolong life without toxic or side effects.

We realize that persisting in taking XZ-C medicine for a longer period of time can help prevent short-term and long-term recurrence and metastasis after radical surgery.

7

About the active ingredients of XZ-C immune regulation anti-cancer Chinese medication

XZ-C1,4 is a compound composed of 28 Chinese herbal medicines. Usually, it is very difficult to extract the total active ingredients of the compound, and the technology is very complicated, and the effective ingredients of the compound are very difficult to extract.

The active ingredients of single medicine can be extracted.

Therefore, except for XZ-C1 which is a decoction of XZ-C series medicines, the rest are all fine powders or capsules of each medicine in order to maintain the independent effective ingredients of each medicine, so as to exert its anti-tumor effect, the powder is a mixture of extremely fine powders, which can maintain the independent effective ingredients of each medicine, and the decoction will cause chemical changes in each medicine, which will inevitably change the effective ingredients composition of each medicine, so it is difficult to know the effective ingredients after decoction. In another words, decoction causes chemical changes in each medicine, which will inevitably change the effective ingredients of each medicine, so it is difficult to know the effective ingredients after decoction.

XZ-C1,4 is a compound composed of 28 Chinese herbal medicines. Usually, it is very difficult to extract the total active ingredients from the compound, the technology is very complicated, and the active ingredients of the compound are difficult to extract.

However, the effective ingredients of the Chinese medications in these XZ-C prescriptions are:

1. *Alkaloids*

2. *Glycosides: Saponins and flavonoid glycosides*

1). Each medicine in the prescription has an anti-tumor active ingredient.

For example, in the prescription, Ganoderma lucidum, its anti-tumor **component A is Ganoderma lucidum polysaccharide**, and its anti-cancer effect is:

Using subcutaneous injection method, in the mice who was transplanted or inoculated with 7 days of S180 ascites carcinoma into the right groin of mice, at a dose of 20 mg/kg, at the 10th day the tumor inhibition rate is 95.6-9 8.5%; for the treatment of leukopenia, the near-term efficiency is 84.6%, and the total number of white blood cells is increased by 1028/mm^3.

The anti-tumor component B of Ganoderma lucidum in the prescription is Fumaric acid. Its anti-tumor effect is that the mice inoculated with S180 are given intragastrically at 60mg/kg, and the tumor weight is weighed 10 days later. The inhibition rate is 37.1% and 38.6%. The weight of the mice does not decrease.

2). Another example is that in the prescription Wintergreen seeds, its anti-tumor component is ursolic acid (Ursolic acid). Its anti-tumor effect is that it has a very significant inhibition rate on liver cancer cells in vitro and can prolong the life of Ehrlich ascites cancer mice.

The pharmacological facts prove that Mingdongqingzi water infusion can inhibit the growth of certain transplanted tumors in animals.

This product **contains oleanolic acid**, which can enhance immune function, increase peripheral leukocytes, enhance the phagocytic ability of reticuloendothelial cells, increase leukopenia caused by chemotherapy or radiotherapy, strengthen the heart, diuresis and protect the liver.

3). Another example is Sophora flavescens in the prescription, its anti-tumor component A is Sophocarpine (Sophocarpine).

Its anti-tumor effect:

In vitro experiments have shown that sophocarpine Ehrlich ascites cancer cells have a direct killing effect: the inhibitory rate of U14, S180, Liol transplantation in mice is 30-60%. It has a certain effect in clinical application.

<u>The anti-tumor component B of Sophora flavescens is Oxyrnatrine (Oxyrnatrine) and its anti-tumor effect</u>:

S180 has significant activity for mice, 500 and 250 ug per day for 5 days,

The tumor weights in the treatment and control groups were 26.1% and 57.9%, respectively.

3. *Another example is the bamboo leaf ginseng in the recipe*:

1). Its anti-tumor component A is ß-Elemene, its anti-tumor effect:

This product has obvious anti-tumor effect on ECA, ARS and other two types of ascites transplanted cancer, and it is also effective for YAS and S180 ascites type.

2). Its anti-tumor component B:

It is the total polysaccharide of ginseng, its anti-tumor effect:

Animal experiments show:

Ginseng total polysaccharide has a stimulating effect on the immune function of the body, and has a significant inhibitory effect on mouse Ehrlich ascites cancer cells at a dose of 400-800mg/kg.

<u>The total polysaccharide of ginseng has no direct killing effect on many tumor cells, and its tumor effect may be due to its adjustment of the body's immune function to enhance the anti-tumor ability of the cancer-bearing host.</u>

3). Its anti-tumor component C is Ginsenoside:

It has a certain inhibitory effect on S180, and its tumor weight inhibition rate is 36.4% at 100, 120 mg/kg/dX7.

a. Ginsenosides can directly act on cancer cells to inhibit their growth;

b. they can also increase the body's resistance to diseases through its metabolic effects and immune regulation, thereby inhibiting tumor growth.

Ginseng acyl extract can inhibit Marine tumor, sarcoma S180, lung cancer-T55.

8

The principles of Formulation for XZ-C prescription

XZ-C1 and XZ-C4 of XZ-C immunomodulatory anti-cancer Chinese medicines are all compound prescriptions, which are in the forms of powders, or capsules. They are a mixture of multi-flavored powders rather than a combination, or instead of a compound, so the active ingredient and pharmacological effect of each flavor exists separately. Therefore, the effective ingredients and pharmacological effects of each drug are separate, in other words, each medicine can be separated separately.

The XZ-C compound is completely different from traditional Chinese medicine decoctions. After A, B, C, D in the traditional compound decoction, the ingredients are completely changed, just like eating "hot pot". The original pharmacological effects of each flavour are lost after decoction, and the original pharmacological effects of each flavour are lost after cooking. It is difficult to know what active ingredients and pharmacological effects are after cooking. In another word, in the traditional compound A, B, C, D, the ingredients are completely changed after boiling, just like eating "hot pot". After boiling together, the original pharmacological effect of each flavor is lost, and the original pharmacological effect of each flavor is lost after cooking. What is the effective ingredient after cooking, it is difficult to know what the pharmacological effect is.

The work of extracting the effective ingredients of the decoction compound is difficult and the technology is very complicated.

And our XZ-C medicine is completely different. It is not decocted, and each flavor is individually ground fine powder, and then mixed in different dosages and packed together (no chemical synthesis). That is, each taste is milled separately, and then mixed together in different doses (no chemical cooperation),

48

The pharmacological effects and active ingredients of each medicine are not changed at all, while the effective ingredients and pharmacological effects of each medicine are retained. This is the reform and innovation of Chinese medicine. In other words, the pharmacological effects and active ingredients of each flavored drug are not changed at all, but the effective components and pharmacological effects of each flavored drug are retained. This is the reform and innovation of traditional Chinese medicine.

Why use a compound prescription instead of a single medicine?

It is because its power is not enough, or insufficient power, and the combined effect of multiple medicines is greater, such as A=a+b+c+d...... Then it must be A>a, A >a+b, A>a+b+c, etc., for example, the tumor inhibition rate of a single flavor is 20%, another flavor is 30%, and another flavor is 31%. Then the tumor inhibition rate of a mixed three flavors may be 20 +30+31, which may reach 81%. Improving immunity, for example, the one flavor is 19%, the second flavor is 40%, and the third flavor is 24%. Then the three flavors together may increase to 83%.

The most important thing is to keep each flavor alone. Each flavor medicine independently exerts its anti-tumor effect and immune-enhancing effect.

In another words, for example, its single-flavor tumor inhibition rate is 20%, another taste is 30%, and another taste is 31%, then the tumor inhibition rate of this three-flavor mixed service once may be 20 + 30 + 31, which may be 81%.

Improving immunity, for example, the first taste is 19%, the second taste is 40%, and the third taste is 24%, then the three tastes may increase to 83% when mixed together. It is the most important to keep each flavor unchanged, and each flavor independently exerts its anti-tumor effect and immunity-enhancing effect.

Furthermore, the compounded and selected principle of XZ-C prescription is to select a prescription according to the biological characteristics of cancer cells and the characteristics of multiple stages and steps of cancer cell metastasis.

Therefore, in the past few years, patients who have taken XZ-C immunoregulatory anti-cancer Chinese medicine for a longer period of time have achieved remarkable results after various cancer surgeries and after radiotherapy in our anti-cancer specialist outpatient clinics with integrated Chinese and Western medicine.

Many patients who are unable to operate at the advanced stage, and are not suitable for radiotherapy or chemotherapy, can also achieve stable disease, control metastasis and spread, improve quality of life, and significantly extend survival after taking XZ-C immunoregulatory Chinese medicine for a long time <u>because each of the XZ-C immune-regulating anti-cancer Chinese medicine has been screened for tumor suppression in solid tumors in tumor-bearing mice twice, for the first time, a single flavor was screened to have a good tumor inhibition rate, for the second time, three indicators were selected for the selection of drugs and prescriptions:</u>

1. It has a good anti-tumor effect;

2. It does not damage normal cells and has no toxic side effects to the body;

3. It can increase immunity. If there is a high tumor inhibition rate, but the immunity is reduced, it cannot be used.

In the newly published book "New Concepts and New Methods of Cancer Treatment", it is clearly stated that after the 16 years of experimental tumor research in our **laboratory** *<u>it is confirmed that the occurrence, development, recurrence, and metastasis of tumors are definitely related to the function of the host's immune organs and the level of immunity.</u>*

<u>It is probable that the drugs which can protect the immune organ and enhance immune function are more important than drugs that suppress or kill cancer cells.</u>

<u>At present, we have realized that traditional anti-cancer drugs are not necessarily anti-metastasis, and anti-metastatic drugs are not necessarily anti-tumor.</u>

The experimental research and clinical verification observation of XZ-C immune regulation and control anti-cancer Chinese medicine show that:

1. It has obvious anti-tumor effect and high tumor inhibition rate;

2. It has a better effect of improving the immune function of the body. Experiments have shown that it can make the thymus of cancerous mice incompletely atrophy (stopping Thymus atrophy) and improve the immune function;

3. It has the function of protecting the hematopoietic system, so that the peripheral white blood cells, platelets and red blood cells after the chemotherapeutic drugs inhibit the bone marrow can be significantly improved;

4. It has a good effect on patients with advanced tumors, can significantly improve the patient's appetite, sleep, physical strength and mental state, can significantly improve symptoms and improve the quality of life;

5. The combined using with chemical medicine in patients who have the advanced cancer has the effect of reducing toxic and side effects, and its curative effect is significantly better than that of chemotherapy alone;

6. Animal experiments have no toxic and side effects. In the 16 years of clinical practice, more than 16,000 patients with advanced cancer have been taking drugs for 3-5 years, and some patients have even been taking drugs for 8-10 years **without any toxic side effects**. Appetite and physical strength are good, and the survival period is significantly prolonged.

9

About the immune function of XZ-C immune regulation and control anti-cancer Chinese medicine on the molecular level

With the continuous deepening of research on traditional Chinese medicine, many traditional Chinese medicines are known to have regulatory effects on the production and biological activity of cytokines and other immune molecules. This is of great significance for elucidating the immunological mechanism of XZ-C regulating anti-cancer Chinese medicine at the molecular level.

(1) **The immune function of T cells enhanced by XZ-C immune regulation and control anti-cancer Chinese medication**

The effective ingredients of XZ-C Chinese medicine include:

(1) Z-C-L

(LBP) can significantly increase the percentage of peripheral blood lymphocytes in mice. Low-dose LBP (5-10mg / kg) can cause lymphocyte proliferation reaction, indicating that LBP can significantly promote proliferation of T cells. Taking 50mg / (kgX d) x 7d as the optimal dose, below this dose there is no obvious promotion effect, and if it exceeds this dose, the effect will decrease instead.

Oral LBP can increase the lymphocyte transformation rate of tumor patients with weak constitution and low white blood cells.

(2) XZ-C4 has the function of regulating the immune system, can activate the T cells in the collective lymph nodes, and stimulate the secretion of hematopoietic growth factors in the T cells. Among the crude drugs that make up XZ-C4, *the hot water extract of rhizome of Atractylodes japonicus has obvious effect of*

stimulating lymph node cells, which is considered to be the basis of XZ-C4 immune regulation.

In another word, among the crude drugs that make up XZ-C4, the rhizome hot water extract of Atractylodes macrocephala has obvious effects on stimulating the aggregation of lymph node cells, *and is considered to be the basis of XZ-C4 immunomodulation.*

(2) **The effect of XZ-C immunoregulatory anti-cancer Chinese medicine on the proliferation, differentiation and hematopoietic function of bone marrow cells**

The active or effective ingredients of XZ-C Chinese medicine include:

(1) **The effect of (1)Z-C-O (PMT) extract (PM-2) and (2) Z-C-Q (LBP) on the proliferation of normal mouse bone marrow hematopoietic stem cells (FPU-S):**

It was to inject PM-2 [50mg/ (kg, d) x 3d] or LBP [10mg/(kg-d) x 3d] into the experimental mice intravenously, and then to kill the testing mice alive on the 9th day.

It was found that in the administration group of the mice, the number of CFU-S in the spleen of mice increased significantly. The number of CFU-S in the PM-2 group and the LBP group were 121% and 136% of the number in the control group, respectively.

Effects on normal mouse bone marrow macrophage colony forming units (colony forming unit of **granulocytes and macrophages, CFU-GM**):

The experimental results show that LBP [5-30mg / (kg · d) x 3d] significantly increases the number of CFU-GM;

PM-2 also significantly enhances the effect of CFU-GM, the effective dose is 12.5-50 mg / (kg · d) x 3d.

CFU-GM mainly consists of granulocyte colonies in the early stage of culture, and the colonies of macrophage cells gradually increase in the future, with macrophage colonies predominant in the later stage.

As can be seen from the above, both PM-2 and LBP have a significant effect on the blood function of normal mice.

And the experiment proves:

In the recovery process of cyclophosphamide from hematopoietic function damage in mice, PM-2 and LBP first stimulated the proliferation of granulocyte progenitor cells, then the bone marrow nucleated cells increased, and finally appeared to promote the recovery of the number of peripheral granulocytes.

(3) Z-C-D (TSPG)

Ginseng total saponins are the effective ingredients of ginseng to promote hematopoietic function.

It can promote:

1). the number *of peripheral red blood cells, hemoglobin and femoral bone marrow cells of myelosuppressive mice,*

2). *increase the division index of bone marrow cells,*

3). stimulate the proliferation of bone marrow hematopoietic cells in vitro,

4). and make them enter the active proliferation cell cycle (S+ G2/M phase).

5). TSPG can promote the proliferation and differentiation of pluripotent hematopoietic stem cells (CFU-S) and myeloid hematopoietic progenitor cells.

6). TSPG can induce the production of hematopoietic growth factor (HGF).

(4) Z-C-H (RGL)

Rehmannia glutinosa can promote:

1). the recovery of RBC and Hb in blood-deficient animals,

2). accelerate the proliferation and differentiation of bone marrow hematopoietic stem cells (CFU-S), and have a significant hematopoietic effect.

3). Continuous injection of Rehmannia glutinosa polysaccharide into mice's abdominal cavity for 6 days can significantly promote the proliferation and differentiation of **hematopoietic stem cells and progenitor cells of** bone marrow in mice,

4). and increase the number of peripheral blood leukocytes.

(5) Z-C-J (ASD)

Polysaccharides have no significant effect on the RBC and Rb of normal mice, but injection of ASD polysaccharides into mice shows significant effects on the proliferation and differentiation of radiation-damaged mouse pluripotent hematopoietic stem cells (CFU-5) and hematopoietic progenitor cells of various lines.

But the decoction has no obvious effect.

(6) Z-C-E(PEW)

The effective part of Yunlingin (small molecule compound extracted from Yunling polysaccharide) can enhance the production of colony stimulating factor (CS F) and increase the level of peripheral blood white blood cells in mice, and can prevent the decrease of white blood cell levels caused by cyclophosphamide. The recovery speed is accelerated, and the effect is stronger than that of sodium ferulate which is the drugs to increase the white cells.

(7) Z-C-Y (PAR)

Its polysaccharide can

1). significantly resist the leukocyte-reducing effect of cyclophosphamide,

2). increase the number of bone marrow cells,

3). promote CSF-induced bone marrow cell proliferation,

4). promote the recovery and reconstruction of hematopoietic function in X-ray irradiated mice,

5). increase hematopoietic stem cells,

6). increase the number of bone marrow cells,

7). and increase white blood cells.

(3) <u>XZ-C immune regulation and control anti-cancer Chinese medicine protects immune organs and increases the weight of immune organs *thymus and spleen*</u>

The active or effective ingredients of XZ-C Chinese medicine include:

(1) Z-C-T (ASD)

Use its extract (equal to 1g per milliliter of the original drug) 15g/kg, 30g/kg and ferulic acid suspension 12.5mg/kg, 25mg/kg to administer the mice every day for 7 consecutive days, all of which can increase significantly Weight of mouse thymus and spleen. Especially in the high-dose group, the effect is more obvious.

Injecting its polysaccharide into the abdominal cavity of mice can also significantly reduce the atrophy of thymus and spleen caused by prednisolone.

(2) Z-C-O (PMT)

PMT6g/ (kgXd) decoction of the extract PM-2 was administered to normal mice for 7 days, which can significantly increase the weight of the thymus and abdominal lymph nodes of the mice, and can antagonize the decrease in the weight of immune organs caused by prednisolone.

Giving 15-month-old mice its decoction (concentration 0.5g/ml) 6g/kg for 14 days can significantly increase the weight and volume of the mouse thymus, thicken the cortex, and increase the cell density.

The combined use of PM and Astragalus can significantly promote the proliferation of non-lymphocytes and help improve the chest microenvironment.

(3) Z-C-W (SCB)

The polysaccharides of SCB can increase the weight of the thymus and spleen in the normal mice.

Gavage with it can also increase the weight of the thymus and spleen of the immunosuppressive mice with cyclophosphamide.

(4) Z-C-M (LLA)

Infusion of LLA decoction to mice for 7 days can significantly increase the weight of thymus and spleen.

(5) Z-C-L

The thymus glands of 15-month-old mice degenerate significantly. Astragalus injection can increase the thymus glands. Under the light microscope, the cortex is significantly thickened and the cell density is significantly increased.

(4) The effect of XZ-C immune regulation and control anti-cancer Chinese medicine on *the activity of LAK cells*

Lymphokine activated killer cells (LAK cells) can be induced by IL-2 cytokines.

Lymph Rokine activated killer cells (Lymph Rokine activated killer cells, LAK cells) can be induced by IL-2 cytokines. LAK cells can kill solid tumor cells that are sensitive and insensitive to NK cells and have a broad-spectrum anti-tumor effect.

The effective ingredients of XZ-C Chinese medicine include:

(1) Z-C-L

AMB polysaccharide can enhance the activity of LAK cells within a certain dose range, with 0.01mg/mi being the strongest, which is three times the killing effect of original LAK cells. If its concentration is too high or too low, it has no effect.

(2) Z-C-U can significantly enhance the activity of spleen LAK cells in tumor-bearing mice to kill tumor cells and increase the activity of red blood cell C3b liquid.

PUPS and IL-2 have a synergistic effect, and can be used as a biological response modifier BRM for LAK/rIL-2 based tumor biological therapy.

(3) Z-C-V

ABB polysaccharides can also enhance the activity of mouse LAK cells and have a significant tumor-inhibiting effect. Its anti-tumor (ABB) mechanism is related to its enhancement of the body's immune function and changes in cell membrane characteristics.

(5) <u>The activity of NK cells enhanced by XZ-C immune regulation and control anti-cancer Chinese medications</u>

Natural killer cells (NK cells) are another type of killer cells in the lymphocytes of humans and mice. They do not require antigen stimulation or antibodies to kill certain cells. It has an important immune function, especially in the body's immune surveillance function. NK cells are the first line of defense against tumors and have a relatively broad anti-tumor spectrum.

NK cells have a broad-spectrum anti-tumor effect, which can kill tumor cells of the same line, the same species and heterogeneity, especially for lymphoma and leukemia cells. NK cells are an important type of immunoregulatory cells. They have a regulatory effect on T cells, B cells, bone marrow stem cells, etc., and they release cytokines (such as IFN-a, IFN-r, IL-2, TNF, etc.) The body's immune function is regulated.

NK cells are an important class of immune regulatory cells, which have regulatory effects on T cells, B cells, bone marrow test stem cells, etc., and through the release of cytokines (such as IFN-a, IFN-r, IL- 2, TNF, etc.) to regulate the body's immune function.

The effective ingredients of XZ-C Chinese medicine include:

(1) XZ-C

Fennel (SDS) can enhance the activity of experimental NK cells. When combined with IL-2, NK activity is more higher. It shows that Fangfeng polysaccharide promotes the activation of NK cells by IL-2 and helps to improve the activity of NK cells.

LBP can enhance the T cell-mediated immune response and NK cell activity in normal mice and cyclophosphamide-treated mice. Intraperitoneal injection of LBP can increase the proliferation of mouse spleen T lymphocytes and enhance the killing function of CTL. The kill rate increased from 33% to 67%.

(2) Z-C-G

Glycyrrhizin (CL) induces IFN in animals and humans, and at the same time enhances NK activity. Clinical experiments by Abe et al. showed that the injection of 80 mg CL in Qingzhengmai increased cell activity by 75% in 21 patients.

Intraperitoneal injection of 0.5 mg/kg GL in mice can enhance the activity of NK cells in the liver.

(3) ZCL (AMB) solution can significantly promote the activity of mouse NK cells in vivo and in vitro, and can directly induce mouse IFN-r (AMB) to process effector cells at a certain concentration (0.1/mI), Cordyceps drunk extract can enhance the activity of mouse NK cells in vivo and in vitro, and can significantly increase the activity of NK cells. 0.5g/kg, 1g/kg, 5g/kg can significantly enhance mouse NK cell activity.

(6) <u>The effect of XZ-C immunomodulatory anticancer Chinese medicine *on interleukin-2 (IL-2)*</u>

The active or effective ingredients of XZ-C Chinese medicine are:

(1) Z-C-T

EBM polysaccharide can significantly enhance the production of human IL-2 at 100ug / ml.

(EBM) shows inhibitory effect at high concentration (2500ug / mI and 5000ug / ml). Or in high concentrations (2500ug/mI and 5000ug/ml), it shows inhibition.

Continuous injection of goat polysaccharide for 7 days can significantly increase the ability of ConA-induced mouse thymus and spleen cells to produce IL-2. Or (EBM) Continuous subcutaneous injection of goat polysaccharide for 7 days can significantly improve the ability of ConA-induced mouse thymus and spleen cells to produce IL-2.

(2) Z-C---Y

PEP sugar has strong immune activity and can promote the production of IL-2. For S180 tumor mice, the IL-2 production ability of mouse spleen cells can be significantly improved.

(3) Z-C--D

Ginseng polysaccharides can significantly promote the induction of IL-2 by peripheral monocytes in healthy patients with nephropathy, and it is in a dose-effect dependent relationship. Or it is dose-dependent.

(7) The inducing and promoting effect of XZ-C immune control and regulation anti-cancer medication on interferon

IFN has broad-spectrum anti-tumor effects and immunomodulatory effects.

IFN can inhibit the proliferation of tumor cells. INF can activate NK cells and CTL to kill tumor cells. At the same time, INF can also cooperate with TNF, IL-1 and IL-2 to enhance the anti-tumor effect.

The effective ingredients in XZ-C immune regulation Chinese medicine include:

(1) Z-C-Z

CVQ polysaccharide 250/kg or 500mg/kg can significantly increase the level of IFN-r produced by mouse splenocytes.

(2) Z-C-D

Ginsenosides (CS) and ginsenosides (PTGS) can

a). induce human whole blood cells; b). monocytes produce IFN-a and IFN-r; and c). can also restore normal IFN-r and IL-2 in tumor-bearing mice.

In the AS H polysaccharide acute lymphocytic leukemia cell line S180 and acute leukemia cell line S7811 the IFN titer produced by polysaccharide stimulation is 5-10 times higher than that of the normal control group.

(3) Z-C-E

Hydromethyl tuckahoe polysaccharide has a variety of physiological activities such as immune regulation, INF induction, indirect anti-virus, and reduction of radiation side effects.

The INF induction kinetics experiment of S180 leukemia cell line with 50mg/mi hydrogen methyl tuckahoe polysaccharide showed that the potency of the HMP at all phases in inducing interferon was significantly higher than that of conventional induction

(4) Z-C-G (GL)

It can induce IFN activity. When mice were injected intraperitoneally with 330 mg/kg GL, the IFN activity reached a peak after 20 hours.

(8) <u>XZ-C immunoregulatory anti-cancer traditional Chinese medicine to promote and *enhance colony stimulating factors* or the promotion and enhancement of colony-stimulating factor by XZ-C immunomodulatory anti-cancer Chinese medication</u>

Colony Stimu latirig Factor (CSF) is a type of low molecular weight glycoprotein that can stimulate the proliferation and differentiation of bone marrow hematopoietic stem cells and various mature blood cells.

The cells that produce CSF include mononuclear phagocytes, T cells, endothelial cells and fibroblasts.

<u>CSF not only participates in the proliferation and differentiation of hematopoietic cells and the regulation of mature cells, but also plays an important role in the host's anti-tumor immunity.</u>

The effective ingredients of XZ-C immunomodulatory Chinese medicine are:

(1). Z-C-Y

PAR polysaccharide can significantly promote the production of CSF and Shangling Polysaccharide II 100---500ug/ml in the spleen cells of experimental mice. It promotes the production of CSF by spleen cells in a dose and time dependent manner. The optimum dose is 100 ug/ml, and the optimum time is 5 days.

Lentinan can also increase the production of CSF.

(2). Z-C-Q

After LBP injection, it can promote the secretion of CSF from mouse spleen and T cells, and increase the activity of serum CSF in mice.

(3). Z-C-T

EDM saponin can significantly promote ConA-induced mouse splenic lymphocyte proliferation and CSF activity.

(9) The role of XZ-C immunomodulatory anti-cancer Chinese medicine to promote tumor necrosis factor (TNF)

Tumor necrosis factor (TNF) is a type of factor that can directly cause tumor cell death.

The main biological effects of TNF are:

Kill or inhibit tumor cells; TNF can kill some tumor cells or inhibit their proliferation both in vivo and in vitro.

The effective ingredients of XZ-C immune regulation Chinese medicine include:

(1) Z-C-Y(PEP)

It can induce TNF production. PEP-1 has an inducing effect on TNF. Inject PEP-180-160mg/kg into the intraperitoneal cavity of mice and seal once every 4 days. Secondly, peritoneal macrophages (PM) must be collected, and 10ug LPS is added to the culture medium. After PM is cultured, the supernatant is taken to determine TNF and IL-1.

It was found that PEP-1 can increase the role of LPS in assisting the production of TNF and IL-1 in parallel. The peak time of induced TNF is the 8th day after two intraperitoneal injections. Compared with the known starter BCG, there is no difference in induced TNF.

(2) Z-C-E

Carboxymethyl tuckahoe polysaccharide (CMP) is the main component extracted from the traditional Chinese medicine tuckahoe.

It can not only enhance the function of mouse spleen cells to produce IL-2 and phagocytes, promote the activity of T, B, NK, LAK cells, but also promote TNF The production.

Experiments prove that CMP is an effective cytokine inducer.

(3) Z-C-Y

ABB polysaccharide can promote ConA-induced TNF-b production in mouse cells, and can also induce mouse peritoneal macrophages to synthesize and secrete

TNF-a, which Achyranthesbidentata Plysaccharzdes(ABP) 20ug/ml stimulates the production of TNF-a and the peak time is 2-6h after the action.

At ABP 100mg/kg, intraperitoneal injection can promote the production of TNF-a, the intensity of the effect is equivalent to BCG (BCG).

(10) The effect of XZ-C immune regulation and control anti-cancer Chinese medication on cell adhesion molecules

Adhesion molecules are mostly glycoproteins, which are distributed on the cell surface or extracellular matrix.

Adhesion molecules play a role in the form of ligand-receptor corresponding, leading to cell-to-cell, cell-to-matrix or cell-matrix-to-cell adhesion, participating in cell information transduction and activation, and stretching and movement of cells, forming thrombosis, and a series of physiological and pathological processes of tumor metastasis.

Intercellular adhesion molecule-i (ICAM-1) is one of the adhesion molecules in the immunoglobulin superfamily.

The effect of XZ-C Chinese medicine on ICAM-1

The effective ingredients of XZ-C Chinese medicine include:

Corn silk, Hobtematiam proved that the ethanol extract of Yushu silk has a significant inhibitory effect on endothelial cell adhesion, and can effectively inhibit the expression of ICAM-1 and TNF, LPS-mediated endothelial cell adhesion activity. In another word, Corn whisker, Hobtematiam proves that the ethanol extract of Yuzhu must significantly inhibit endothelial cell adhesion, and can effectively inhibit ICAM-1 expression and TNF, LPS-mediated endothelial cell adhesion activity.

10

About the anti-tumor ingredients; the structural formula; the existence location; the anti-tumor effect of XZ-C immune regulation and control anti-cancer Chinese medication

1. **XZ-Cl-C SNL**

Anti-tumor component A:
Vitamin A / Vitamin A
The structural formula:

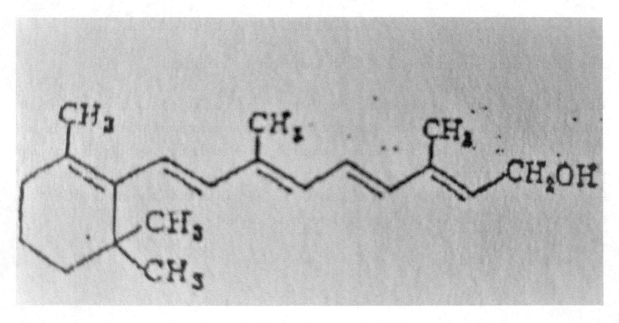

The existing part:

It is the whole plant of this plant and its content is 9666IU%

(% of international units)

<u>The antitumor effect:</u>

V_A has a certain anti-tumor activity.

1). Wald did a research study from 1975 to 1979, which showed that V_A has an anti-tumor effect in the body;

2). **Bontwell found that V_A can block the accumulation of mucopolysaccharides in the cell membrane caused by the action of carcinogens.**

3). **And it can block receptors that can bind to carcinogens.**

<u>**A new method of tumor treatment:**</u>

Normal glycosides plus LETS (large extracellular metastatic sensitive protein), in which the synthesis of both substances is affected by V_A, which shows the importance of V_A in the treatment of cancer.

At the same time, V_A and its derivatives can ***reverse*** cancerous cells after the induction of chemical carcinogens, virus induction and ionizing radiation.

2. Antitumor component B in XZ-Cl-C SNL:
<u>**Vitamin C**</u>
The structural formula:

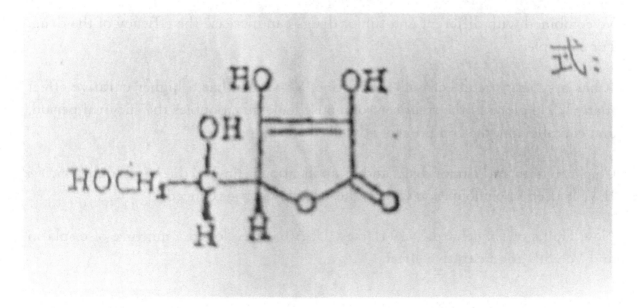

The existing parts:

It is the whole plant of this plant and its content is 20mg%.

The antitumor effect:

1. Vc acts as an anti-oxidant in the anti-tumor effect, blocking the synthesis of carcinogenic nitroso compounds in the body by succinic acid salts and several amines.

Canieron applied Vc at 10g / day for 100 tumor patients for a long-term, which was 42 times more effective than in the control group, and had better efficacy in gastrointestinal cancer.

Murata applied high-dose Vc to treat cervical cancer which is 5.7 times more effectively than small-dose.

Kihstratos caused sarcoma growth in rats with benzoxanthene, and then gave a large amount of Vc to the treatment group, indicating that Vc has the effect of inhibiting the growth and occurrence **of sarcoma.**

It also has top protection against bladder cancer and skin cancer. Epidemiological tumor incidence is also related to Vc intake.

Vc combined with different anti-tumor drugs can increase the efficacy of the drug. For example:

It has a synergistic effect with vincristine. Vc+CCNu has a higher curative effect than CCNu alone in the treatment of mouse leukemia, doubles the survival period, and can alleviate the condition of advanced cancer patients.

Cisplatin is an anti-tumor drug, and its application is limited due to its high toxicity. If Vc is used in combination with it, the toxicity can be reduced.

Now Hollis of Englehard, New Jersey, USA has developed a mixture of cisplatin and Vc with good curative effect.

The whole plant contains Solasonine and Solanine which are also active against SI80 sarcoma. The whole plant contains solanine (Solasonine) and solanine (solanine) also have activity on SI80 sarcoma.

The total alkaloids of Solanum vulgare extracted from dried green fruits of Solanum radiata have an inhibitory rate of 40-50% on animal transplantation tumors.

In tissue culture, the total alkali concentration of Solanum is 50-500mcg/ml, it can inhibit the growth of meningioma cells after it works for 24h.

The alkaline component isolated from the total alkali of Solanum has the strongest anti-cancer activity and has obvious cytotoxic effect. The concentration is 10mcg/ml. After 15h, HeLa cells can be disintegrated. Its extract also has a certain inhibitory effect on mouse sarcoma 180 ascites.

Solamine can also be used as a stimulant for the hematopoietic system and has the effect of increasing white blood cells.

It can be used with Scutellaria barbata and Lithospermum to treat malignant hydatidiform mole with better effect.

Cooperate with surgical resection, chemotherapy, radiotherapy for uterine choriocarcinoma, ovarian cancer, liver cancer and other cases, it also achieved varying degrees of effects.

This product has an inhibitory effect on mouse cervical cancer U14, sarcoma S180, Ehrlich ascites carcinoma and mouse lymphosarcoma。

This product is administered to mice inoculated with Ehrlich ascites carcinoma, lymphocytic leukemia L615, sarcoma S180 and other tumors, which can inhibit the above tumor strains.

<u>Animal in vivo tests</u> have an inhibitory effect on gastric cancer cells.

<u>In vitro experiments using the methylene blue test tube method </u>it showed that it has an inhibitory effect on tumor cells (leukemia).

SNL base has anti-cancer cell nuclear division effect. The total base of SNL extracted from the dried green fruits of this product can inhibit the transplantation tumor of animals by 40% -50%.

In tissue culture, the total alkali concentration of SNL is 50-500ug / ml, which can inhibit the growth of brain tumor cells in the time of 24 hours.

3. Z-Cl-B SLT
Anti-tumor ingredients:
ß-Solamarine
The structural formula:

The effective part:
SLT whole grass
The antitumor effect:

The whole plant has an anti-tumor effect. It has been used as a folk medicine to treat cancer in many countries in the world for a long time. **P-Solamarine is its active ingredient**. At a dose of 30 mg / kg, it can make that the tumor weight of mouse sarcoma 180 from 1285 mg reduce to 274mg of the control group, its inhibition rate was 78.6%. Or 30mg / kg of its amount can make the tumor weight of mouse sarcoma 180 from 1285mg reduce to 274mg in the control group.

The whole grass has anti-cancer effects **on human lung cancer**.

Recently, it has been reported that anti-tumor active ingredients which are extracted from SLT to make health foods have a certain anti-tumor effect and are almost non-toxic.

SLT also contains Australian Solanine which has inhibitory activity **on mouse sarcoma 180**.

It has been reported recently:

The effective anti-tumor ingredients which are obtained or extracted from SLT with water or water-soluble organic solvents or mixed solvents **can be made into oral or parenteral medicine**. The dosage is 1g / d for oral administration and 60mg / d for parenteral administration.

The drug can inhibit various tumors, such as **sarcoma S-180, human neck cancer cells,** etc., and its toxicity is extremely low. Murakami Kotaro et al. isolated two steroidal glycosides from SLT, each with a certain anti-tumor effect.

SLT has an inhibitory effect on subcutaneous inoculation of <u>mouse sarcoma S 180, cervical cancer U14, and Ehrlich ascites carcinoma.</u>

1). In vitro experiments, the hot water extract of this product inhibited <u>human cervical cancer cell JTC-26</u> by 100%. **It has no effect on normal cells.**

2). **In vivo tests, the inhibition rate of mouse sarcoma S$_{180}$ was 14.57%.**

This product contains an effective anti-cancer ingredient ß- solanine, which has a significant inhibitory effect on mouse sarcoma S180 and human *mouse Wacker cancer W256.*

4.XZ-Cl-A ApL
1). Anti-tumor ingredients:
<u>Agrimonniin</u>

2). The active part:
<u>The whole plant for this plant</u>

3). Antitumor effect:
a. Okucla and other scholars have isolated agrimonniin from ApL grass, which it has been proved that agrimoniin is the main component of anti-cancer in this plant Apl.

b. Before and after inoculation **of MM2 breast cancer cells**, this product is given 10mg / kg ip. As a result, all tumors were rejected, and either PO or ip administration could prolong the survival period of tumor-bearing animals.

c. Agrimonniin can also inhibit the growth **of MH134 liver cancer and Meth-A cellulose sarcoma**.

d. In the medium with or without calf serum, MM2 breast cancer cells and Agrimonniinn are treated for 2h, and then cultured in a humidified CO_2 incubator at 37^0C for 48h.

It was found that when calf serum was not added, Agrimonniin showed a strong cytotoxic effect on MM_2 cells, and its IC_{50} was 2.66ug/ml. But adding bovine fetal serum to the medium, the effect is reduced to about 4% of the original, that is, IC_{50} is 62.5% ug/ml.

e. After intraperitoneal injection of agrimonniin for 4 days, the uptake rate of H3-thymidine in MM2 breast cancer and MH134 liver cancer cells was significantly inhibited.

<u>These results indicate that agrimonniin is a strong anti-tumor tannic acid, and its anti-tumor effect may be due to the enhancement of the host's immune response by the drug acting on tumor cells and certain immune cells.</u>

ApL grass adopts water extraction and alcohol precipitation method to make a 1:1 (1g crude drug/ml) solution with pH 6.5. Use this preparation to test inhibit S_{180}, cervical cancer U_{14}, brain tumor B_{22}, Ehrlich ascites cancer EAC, black Cord tumor B10, rat Wacker carcinoma W256, etc.

The results show that it has a good inhibitory effect on the above transplanted tumors, and the inhibition rates are between 36.2-65.9%, and the P values are all less than 0.05, which is a significant difference.

ApL grass water extract has a strong inhibitory effect on human cancer cells JTC-26 in vitro, with an inhibition rate of 100% and a growth promotion effect on normal cells of 100%.

Daily intraperitoneal injection of ApL oxalol injection 30mg / kg has an obvious experimental therapeutic effect on sarcoma S_{37} and murine cervical cancer U_{14}, with a tumor growth inhibition rate of 47% and 38.7%. Rats were administered at a dose of 0.625g / day, the inhibition rate was 47.4%, and the inhibition rate for liver cancer solid type was 52.6%.

It was to extract liver cancer ascites fluid and to dilute it with sterilized physiological water to (1-2) x10^7 cancer cells per ml. Then it was inoculated into mice, each mouse was intraperitoneally injected with 0.2ml. The control group was injected with the same amount of saline,

It is to observe the death time of each mouse within 30 days, and calculate the life extension rate for the undead.

The results:

24 animals in the treatment group survived for an average of (26.2±0.9) days, and the control group survived for an average of (17.5±1.3) days. The life extension rate was 49.6%.

Apl oxafol has a significant life-prolonging effect on animals with liver cancer and ascites cancer.

5.Z-C-D PGS
Antitumor component A:
ß-Elemene
Structural formula:

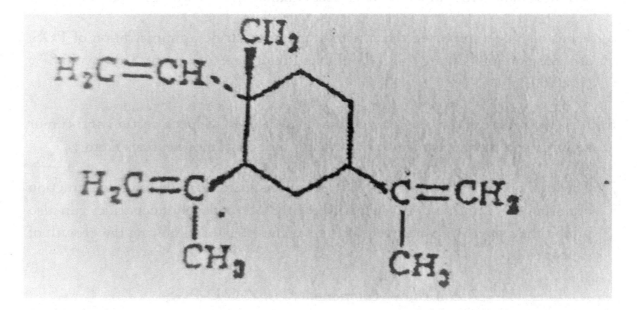

The existing parts:

It is in volatile oil of the root and about 10% in the flowers

The antitumor effect:

This product has obvious anti-tumor effect on ECA, ARS and other two types of ascites transplanted animal tumors, and it is also effective for S180 ascites.

6. Antitumor component B in Z-C-D PGS:
PGS total polysaccharides;
Antitumor effect:

Animal experiments show that:

1). PGS total polysaccharides have a stimulating effect on the body's immune function.

2). It has a certain inhibitory effect on the transplanted tumor S180 in mice.

3). It has a significant inhibitory effect on mice Ehriich ascites cancer cells when dosed at 400-800mg / kg.

4). PGS total polysaccharide has no direct killing effect on many tumor cells, and its anti-tumor effect may be due to its adjustment of the body's immune function, so that it makes the tumor-bearing host enhance the anti-tumor ability.

5). It has also been reported that the total polysaccharide administration of PGS, at a dose of 460.620 mg / kg / d, inhibited the tumor weight of S180 by 76.81% (P <0.001).

6). It is also reported that the total polysaccharide of PGS has a certain anti-tumor activity, and the mechanism may be that it induces tumor necrosis factor;

7). The total polysaccharide of PGS can enhance and activate the immune function of normal mice and tumor-bearing mice. 8). PGS total polysaccharides can also inhibit the growth of cancer cells. Or it has the effect of inhibiting the growth of cancer cells.

7. Antitumor component C in Z-C-D PGS
PGS saponin Ginsenoside
The structural formula: (general formula)

The antitumor effect:

1). It has an obvious inhibitory effect on mouse sarcoma-180. At 100, 120mg / kg / dx7, the tumor weight inhibition rate is 60%, 48%;

2). For mice with Ehrlich ascites carcinoma (ECS) at a dose of 100 mg / kg / dx70, the inhibiting rate is 36%, 40%;

3). For S-180 at a dose of 100 mg / kg / dx 10, the inhibition rate was 41-61% (P <0.05);

4). The large doses also had a certain anti-tumor effect on U_{14}.

When used in combination with the chemotherapy drug cyclophosphamide, it can enhance the anti-tumor effect of the chemotherapy drug.

Its anti-tumor effect is more complicated:

First, it can <u>directly</u> act on cancer cells to inhibit their growth or reverse them.

Second, it can also increase the body's resistance to disease through the effects of metabolism and regulation of immune function, thereby inhibiting the growth of tumors.

Clinical trials or experiments at the country and abroad proved:

It has a therapeutic effect on gastric cancer, which not only reduces the tumor size, but also increases appetite, improves the body's immunity, and prolongs the patient's survival time.

PGS saponin as an anti-tumor agent for the human body has a wide range of adaptation and almost no side effects.

The scope of adaptation is gastric cancer, rectal cancer, breast cancer, uterine cancer, oral cancer, esophagus cancer, gallbladder cancer, kidney tumor, lung cancer, brain tumor, liver cancer, skin cancer, etc., which it almost has effect for all tumors.

Method of administration:

1). *It can be taken orally, at 100-300 mg / day. The medicine can be given by separately 2-3 times.*

2). *1-10% hydrophilic ointment or hydrophobic ointment can also be used for external use.*

a. The report by Ruan Shi from the Korea Atomic Energy Research Institute:

In experimental animals treated with carcinogens, long-term oral administration of red ginseng can reduce the incidence of tumors and inhibit tumor growth.

b. Odashima and other reports:

Using cultured liver cancer cells to study the effect of PGS saponins on liver cancer cells, it was found that PGS can cause structural changes in cancer cells, indicating that PGS cells can induce **cancer cells to reverse**.

c. Hiroshi Abe and other reports:

PGS saponins has a certain effect on inducing **the reversal** of liver cancer cells.

d. Li Xianggao believes:

PGS saponin Rnl can inhibit 3-O-methyl glucose in liver cancer cells from overflowing through the cell membrane, so it is speculated that the inhibitory effect of PGS saponin Rnl on membrane transport may be non-specific.

In addition to the research on the anti-tumor activity of **ginseng root saponins**, the tumor inhibitory effect of ginseng **flower saponins** has also been reported:

Scholars such as Yu Yongli used Jilin ginseng flower total saponins to study the effect of NKC-INF-IL-2 regulatory network and its anti-tumor effect.

The results show that:

PGS flower total saponins can promote the natural killing effect (NKC) of rat spleen, and can induce interferon (γ-IFN) and interleukin (IL-2) under Con-A formation. The body can increase the NKC activity of normal mice, and enhance the NKC activity and the ability to produce γ-IFN and IL-2 in mice with transplanted tumors. It shows that PGS floral saponins play a normal regulatory role on the NKC-IFN-IL-2 regulatory network, and exert a wide range of immunological effects through this regulatory network.

Liang Zhongpei's application of PGS whiskers on dimethyl cream yellow induced liver cancer in rats.

the result shows:

PGS whisker syrup can increase the percentage of ANAE-positive lymphocytes, which is a reduction in the incidence of liver cancer, a smaller mass, and a higher degree of cancer cell differentiation. Fibrous tissue hyperplasia and lymphocyte infiltration around the cancer focus indicate that PGS whisker syrup can promote cellular immunity It can prevent or control liver cancer induced by chemical carcinogens.

Liang Zhongpei and others applied PGS whisker to the effect of dimethyl butter yellow-induced liver cancer in rats.

The results show:

PGS whisker syrup can increase the percentage of ANAE-positive lymphocytes. It is to reduce the incidence of liver cancer is reduced, the tumor is smaller, the degree of differentiation of cancer cells is higher, and there are fibrous tissue proliferation and lymphocyte infiltration around the cancer focus, indicating that PGS whisker syrup can promote the body's cellular immunity Function, prevent or control liver cancer induced by chemical carcinogens

Ginseng has inhibitory effects on various experimental animals.

Long-term feeding of ginseng in rats and mice can reduce the incidence of tumors and inhibit tumor growth in lung adenomas caused by aflatoxin and lung cancer induced by uratan in mice.

The main active ingredient of ginseng's anti-tumor effect is ginsenoside.

Among them, ginsenoside Rg3 can strongly inhibit the formation of new tumor organs, inhibit tumor recurrence, spread and metastasis, and inhibit melanoma and S180 solid tumors in mice by 60%, and inhibit lung metastasis and liver metastasis of various animal and human tumors. The rate is 60%-70%.

Ginsenoside Rg3 is promising as an anti-metastatic agent.

8. Z-C-E PCW
The antitumor component A
<u>Adenine</u>

The structural formula:

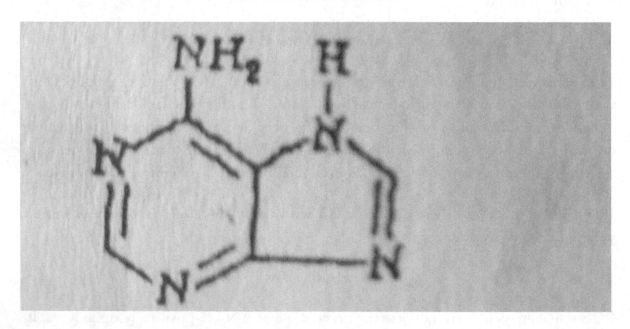

The existing parts:

There is in the sclerotium of the plant or in the sclerotia of plants

Antitumor effect:

It is used to prevent and treat leukopenia caused by various reasons, especially due to tumor chemotherapy, radiotherapy and benzene poisoning. Its phosphate can stimulate leukocyte proliferation. Leukocyte proliferation is generally seen about 2-4 weeks after medication. Using this product before or at the same time of tumor chemotherapy can prevent the occurrence of leukopenia, so it can extend the chemotherapy time.

9. Antitumor component B in Z-C-E PCW:

Pachyma

The structural formula

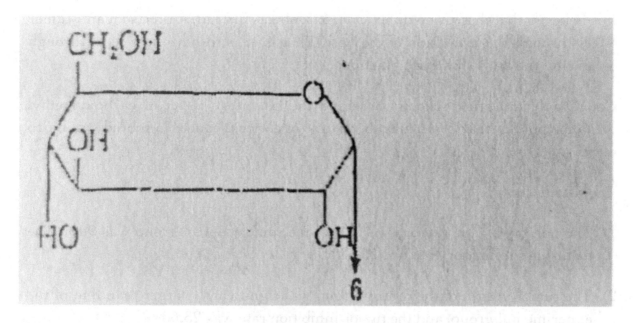

The antitumor effect:

The reserch shows:

New pachyman polysaccharide (pachyman):

1. The pachyman structure was slightly modified in 1970 by Chihara and others, that is, the ß (1-6) side chain was removed and it was formed and synthised.

Pachymaran has obvious antitumor activity, but poor water solubility.

2. Carboxymethyl-pachymaran (Carboxymethyl-pachymaran) was synthesized by Hamuro et al. in 1971 by carboxymethylating pachymaran. It shows obvious anti-tumor activity in animal experiments.

Hamuro, J and other experiments proved:

Pachyman Bio-New Poria Polysaccharides, CM-pachymaran, HM-pachyman 2-4, have obvious anti-tumor activity.

Moreover, the anti-tumor activity has a great relationship with its dosage and route of administration, and the optimal dosage of the appropriate route of administration must be selected.

There are also reports on the anti-tumor mechanism of pachyman and its derivatives:

It is believed that there is no direct cytotoxic effect. Instead, it exerts an anti-tumor effect through the mediation of the host. That is, it is to have its effects through enhancing the body's immune function.

Cao Qiaoli and other scholars observed the inhibitory effect of carboxymethyl tuckahoe polysaccharide on lung metastasis of cervical cancer in inbred strain 615 mice.

The results show

1). The non-metastatic rate was 64%, and the tumor control group was 94%. The metastasis inhibition rate was 75.68%.

2). The tumor weight of the control group was significantly larger than that of the experimental group, and the tumor inhibition rate was 23.58%.

The above results indicate that carboxymethyl tuckahoe polysaccharides do have certain anti-cancer activity.

<u>There are also reports at home and abroad:</u>

<u>Carboxymethyl tuckahoe polysaccharide is a good immune enhancer and is used to treat a variety of tumors.</u>

US Patent 4339435 reports:

The sclerotium of Poria cocos is artificially cultured to obtain mycelium, and then this mycelium is extracted with water or a water-soluble organic solvent such as ethanol to obtain an anti-cancer drug "A-1", which not only has good anti-cancer activity, Moreover, it is non-toxic and has an inhibition rate of 92% against S180. This anti-cancer substance accounts for 24.2% of the cultured mycelium.

Xu Jin et al. reported that a group of fat-soluble tetracyclic triterpene organic acids were isolated from Poria cocos, collectively referred to as Poria cocos, which have obvious inhibitory effects on Ehrlich ascites carcinoma and S180, and also have a certain effect on the metastasis of Lewis lung cancer in mice. Combined with anti-cancer drugs such as cyclophosphamide, it has a certain synergistic effect, and tests have proved that Poria cocos has an immune-enhancing effect.

In 1986, the Japanese scholar Jiufan Jinshan isolated a water-soluble anti-tumor polysaccharide from artificially cultured Poria mycelium, called Poria polysaccharide H11, which accounted for about 0.6% of the dried mycelium, and used it at 4 mg/kg. Injected into ICR/TCL mice subcutaneously for 10 consecutive days, the inhibition rate of S180 (solid type) reached 94%. This report shows that there are polysaccharides in Poria cocos that have anti-tumor activity without structural modification.

It has also been reported that the ß-Pachyman contained in Poria cocos is treated with drugs and methods to obtain Poria cocosant complex (U-P for short), which has obvious anti-tumor effect, and its inhibition rate is 57%. It can prolong the survival period of tumor-bearing mice, increase the spleen index, and have a direct effect on tumor cells.

Wu Bo and other scholars have also conducted experimental studies on the anti-tumor effect and mechanism of Poria cocos polysaccharide (PPS) to observe the effect of Poria cocos polysaccharide (PPS) on the proliferation of mouse S180 cells and human leukemia K562 cells in vitro.

It was found that PPS has a strong inhibitory effect on the proliferation of the two kinds of cells. In order to explore its anti-tumor mechanism, the composition of the S180 cell membrane was analyzed. The results showed that the PPS contacted the cells for 24 hours, causing the cell membrane sialic acid content to increase and the membrane phospholipid content to decrease, but membrane cholesterol content, membrane fluidity and membrane neutral fatty acid composition are not affected.

The PPS and S180 cell membranes were developed together under appropriate conditions, and it was found that the influence of PPS to interfere with the inositol phospholipid metabolism of the membrane is an important link.

There are also some reports on the changes in the anti-tumor mechanism and biochemical properties of PPS.

Poria cocos (PPS) has a significant irreversible inhibitory effect on the DNA synthesis of mouse leukemia L1210 cells, and the inhibitory effect increases with increasing dose.

Poriatin has a synergistic effect on anticancer drugs:

The tumor suppressor rate (mouse sarcoma S180) used in combination with mitomycin was 38.9% (5-Pu alone was 38.6%);

For mouse leukemia L1210, the life extension rate of cyclophosphamide alone is 70%, and the combined use of poriarin and trifacrine is 168.1%.

Dethymic mice proved that the anti-tumor effect of PPS is related to the thymus.

Fungal polysaccharides can non-specifically stimulate the function of the reticuloendothelial system, improve the host's immunity against cancer cell-specific antigens, and achieve cancer resistance.

Poria Polysaccharide and Poria cocos has obvious anti-tumor effect. It can inhibit the growth of mouse solid tumor S180 and prolong the survival time of Ehrlich ascites cancer mice. Poria polysaccharides have a significant effect on the proliferation of mouse ascites sarcoma S180 cells and human chronic myelogenous leukemia K562 cells cultured in vitro.

The anti-tumor mechanism of Poria cocos polysaccharides includes two ways of improving the host's immune system and direct cytokine effects.

The anti-tumor mechanism of Poriacin may be to inhibit tumor cell DNA synthesis by inhibiting the nucleoside transport of tumor cells, and increase the ability of macrophages to produce tumor necrosis factor (TNF), and enhance the effect of killing tumor cells.

Intraperitoneal injection of carboxymethyl pachymaran (PPS) 5-200mg/kgxd for 100 consecutively, the groups above 10mg have a significant inhibitory effect on S180.

Inhibition of mouse sarcoma S180 and Ehrlich ascites carcinoma (EAC) and oral administration, 8 days, can increase tumor necrosis factor (TNF) level in tumor-bearing mice and significantly increase the activity of natural killer (NK) cells.

Giving mice carboxymethyl tuckahoe polysaccharide (250mg/kg.d) for 25 days has a significant inhibitory effect on the lung metastasis of cervical cancer U14.

The sarcoma S180 cells were inoculated subcutaneously in ICR/JCL mice, and 24 hours later, the intraperitoneal injection of carboxymethyl tuckahoe polysaccharide, 5mg/kg dose, once a day for 10 days, the results showed that the poria tuckahoe polysaccharide tumor inhibition rate was 95%.

Carboxymethyl tuckahoe polysaccharide has a strong inhibitory effect on mouse inhibitory tumor U_{14}.

Using 500mg/kg, 100mg/kg, 50mg/kg doses for the test, the results of the tumor inhibition rates were 75.5%, 92.7%, 78.7%, of which the 100 mg/kg dose was the best.

The 10-day survival period of mice inoculated with Ehrlich's ascites cancer by continuous intraperitoneal injection of carboxymethyl tuckahoe polysaccharide (100mg/kg.d) was 23.49% longer than that of the control group. The amount of ascites was reduced by 7%, and the total number of cancer cells was reduced by 139.20%. The results of the test on the effect of 3H thymidine (3 H-TdR) incorporation into cancer cells have been shown. PPS can inhibit DNA synthesis of Ehrlich ascites cancer cells.

The anti-tumor effect of PPS is related to the dose. The anti-tumor test was carried out with PPS, using 3 different doses of 100mg/kg, 50mg/kg, and 5mg/kg. The results showed that the tumor suppression rates were 92.3%, 96.1%, and 53.4%, respectively.

10. Z-Cl--G GuF
Antitumor component A:
Glycyrrhiza acid
The structural formula:

The existing parts:
The roots and rhizomes of this plant.
Antitumor effect:

This product can produce morphological changes on rat ascites liver cancer and mouse Ehrlich ascites carcinoma (EAC) cells, and has an inhibitory effect on Yoshida's sarcoma subcutaneously suppressed.

Monoammonium glycyrrhetate, namely glycyrrhetinate, is made from glycyrrhizin as raw material, which has inhibitory effect on mouse Ehrlich water ascites carcinoma sarcoma.

At the same time, glycyrrhizinate has a certain detoxification effect on some highly toxic anticancer drugs.

For example, a natural product with a certain anti-tumor effect: Camptothecirie causes a toxic reaction and limits the use of drugs. Glycyrrhizinate not only does not reduce its efficacy when reducing the toxicity of camptothecin, but also has a certain synergistic effect. In animal experiments, the use of camptothecin caused a decrease in the number of white blood cells in mice. Glycyrrhizinate has a protective effect.

The hot water extract of this product has an inhibitory rate of 70%-90% on human cervical cancer cells JTC-26.

11. Antitumor component B in Z-Cl—G GuF:

Giycyrrhetinic aicd

The structural formula:

The existing parts:

The roots and rhizomes of the original plant

Antitumor effect:

Glycyrrhetinic acid has an inhibitory effect on Oberling-Guerin myeloma transplanted in rats. Its sodium salt has an inhibitory effect on the growth of Ehrlich ascites carcinoma and sarcoma-45 cells in mice, and it is effective even if taken orally.

12. Anti-tumor component C in XZ-Cl-G GiF
Liguirtin
Structural formula:

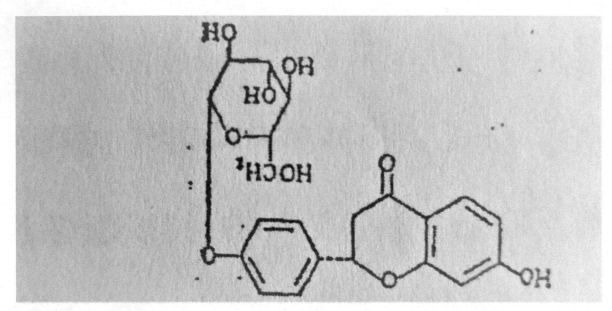

The existing parts:
The root of this plant.
Antitumor effect:

This product has an inhibitory effect on the changes in the morphology of rat ascites liver cancer and mouse Ehrlich ascites cancer cells. It also has anti-tumor effect. It has an inhibitory effect on rat breast tumors.

It has a preventive effect on rat gastric cancer and can reduce the incidence of gastric cancer.

In addition, glycyrrhizin can significantly inhibit aflatoxin B1 to induce precancerous lesions of liver.

13. Z--C-K LwF
Anti-tumor ingredients:
Tetramethylpyrazine (TTMP)
Anti-tumor effect:

1. It is reported in the literature that TTMP can inhibit the activity of TXA2 synthase.

2. Li Xuetang and others reported:

One-time administration of TTMP has a certain anti-metastatic effect on the metastasis of liver cancer cells in mice.

3. Liu Jinrong and others reported TTMP anti-tumor effect and its mechanism. The experimental results show:

TTMP administered at a dose of 20 mg/day for 18 days can significantly inhibit the artificial lung metastasis of B16-F10 melanoma. The isotope incorporation method determines that TTMP can enhance the activity of NK cells in the spleen of normal and tumor-bearing mice. And it can antagonize the inhibitory effect of cyclophosphamide on NK cell activity.

The anti-tumor metastasis effect of TTMP may be related to the reduction of plasma TXB content in mice and the enhancement of NK cell activity.

4. Some scholars also reported:

Adenine is isolated from this plant, and its pharmacological activity has been confirmed. It can stimulate leukocyte proliferation and prevent leukopenia, especially for leukopenia caused by solid radiotherapy or chemotherapy.

TTMP has a certain anti-metastasis effect on mouse liver cancer cells.

14.Z-C--LAMB

Antitumor component B:
b-Sitosterol
Structural formula:

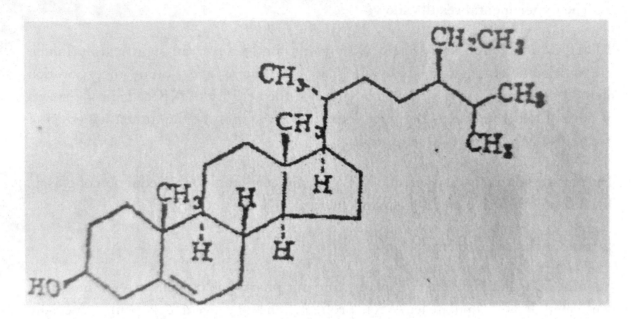

Existing part: in the root of the plant.
Anti-tumor effect:

1). b-Guzitol has marginal activity for lymphocytic leukemia p134;

2). it has activity for mouse adenocarcinoma 715, and its inhibitory tumor weight (TWI) is 58%;

3). It is only active for mouse Lewis lung cancer, and its tumor weight (TWI)>58%;

4). it has inhibitive effect for rat WACKER tumor 256, and its tumor weight (TW1)>58%.

There are reports:

A certain amount of polysaccharides is contained in the root of AMB, and the content of AMB polysaccharide is 1.34%-2.04%, which is composed of several polysaccharides.

It has a wide range of biological activities and has anti-tumor effects in in vivo experiments, but in vitro experiments cannot directly kill cancer cells, indicating that AMB polysaccharides work by enhancing immune function.

AMB can increase the cAMP content in human and mouse plasma, inhibit tumor growth, and even reverse tumor cells.

It can promote the increase of animal white blood cells;

It can combat human leukopenia caused by chemotherapy or radiotherapy;

It can promote the body's immune function;

It can suppress and kill tumor cell tumors.

The hot water extract was tested in vivo and the inhibition rate of mouse sarcoma 180 was 41.7%. The alcohol extract is invalid.

At present, AMB is commonly used clinically as an anti-cancer and righting medicine.

Zhou Shuying and others reported the anti-tumor experimental research of AMB polysaccharide:

1). The results of in vivo experiments show that:

Intramuscular injection of APS 2.5 mg/kg, 5 mg/kg, 10 mg/kg, 20 mg/kg four doses has a significant inhibitory effect on the transplanted tumor S180 liver cancer in mice.

2). The in vitro test results show:

The compatibility of APS and interleukin 2 can significantly increase the killing rate of LAK cells to target cells P851 and Y ac-1 cells. Its anti-tumor mechanism is related to its increase in immune function.

3). In vivo test, the inhibitory rate of AMB hot water extract on mouse sarcoma S180 is 41.7%.

The inhibitory rate of human lung adenocarcinoma SPC-A-I cell proliferation index was 12.25%.

In the process of inducing lung cancer in rats with MCA lipiodol solution, the tumor suppression test with MCA injection showed that the cancer rate of the drug group was 16.28%, and the cancer rate of the control group was 51.52%. The difference between the two groups was very significant.

4). MCA has a certain inhibitory effect on DNA synthesis of human ovarian cancer cells. When the concentration of the drug increases, the inhibitory effect is also enhanced; the prolonged drug action time, the inhibitory effect on tumor cell DNA synthesis is also enhanced. Or the prolonged action time of the drug also enhanced the inhibition of tumor cell DNA synthesis.

5). MCA polysaccharide has a synergistic effect on the activation of T lymphocytes in cancerous ascites.

15. Z-C-M LIA
Anti-tumor ingredients:
Ursolic acid
Structural formula:

It is existing parts:
In the leaves of the plant
Anti-tumor effect:

a. In vitro cancer cell culture it has a very significant inhibition rate; it can prolong the life of mice with ascites cancer.

b. Pharmacological experiment proves or Pharmacological test certificate:

c. This product water infusion can inhibit the growth of certain transplanted tumors in animals.

d. In vitro screening it has a certain inhibitory effect on tumor cells.

e. It has a certain enhancement effect on the body's immune function;

f. It has the effect of increasing the white blood cells caused by chemotherapy and radiotherapy.

g. It has also been reported that the active ingredient in this product for raising white blood cells is zidenolicacid.

16. Z-C--N CzR
Anti-tumor component A:
Curcumol
The structural formula:

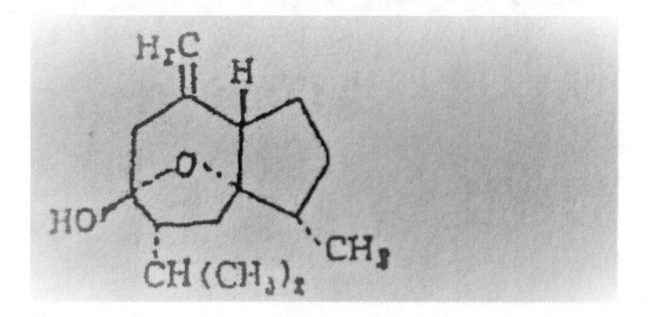

The existing part:
the rhizome of the plant.
Anti-tumor effect:

Curcumol has anti-tumor effects.

1. For mouse sarcoma S37, the inhibition rate of 75mg/kg dose is 53.47-61.96%;

2. At a dose of 75mg/kg, the inhibition rate for mouse cervical cancer U14 was 45.1-77.13%;

3. At the same dose, the inhibition rate of Ehrlich ascites carcinoma (EAC) in mice was 65.8-78.9%.

4. It is clinically used for the treatment of cervical cancer with good curative effect.

17. Z-C--N CzR
Anti-tumor component B:

Curdione

The structural formula:

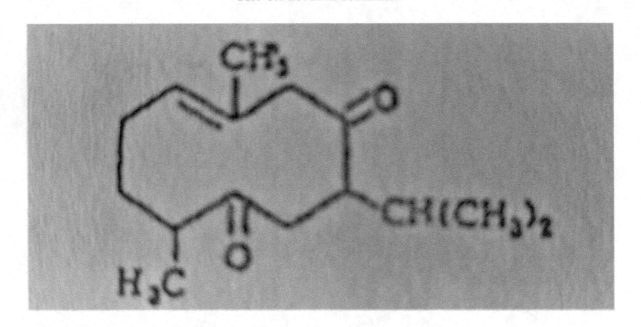

The existing part:

It is the rhizome of the plant.

Anti-tumor effect:

Turmeric dione has a significant inhibitory effect on mouse sarcoma 37, mouse apical carcinoma U14 and mouse Ehrlich ascites carcinoma, and can cause cancer cells to degenerate and die.

Ehrlich ascites carcinoma treated with this product can successfully make mice gain active immunity. The clinical results show that it has a good effect on cervical cancer.

There are also reports:

ß-elemenc is isolated from the same genus of Curcurna wenyuj in Y.H. Chen.et C Ling. This product also has certain anti-cancer activity.

Experiments show that ß-elemene can significantly prolong the survival time of mice with Ehrlich ascites carcinoma and ascites reticulosarcoma.

It has a strong killing effect on liver cancer cells cultured in vitro;

It can also significantly reduce the nucleic acid content of Ehrlich ascites cancer cells, especially the reduction of RNA content is more important.

The effects of ß-elemene on leukocytes and bone marrow nucleated cells and immune test:

The test results show that ß-elemene has relatively low toxicity.

100% Curcuma injection 0.3-0.5ml injected into the abdomen of mice has a good effect on sarcoma S180. The inhibition rate is above 50%.

Using crystal 1 (curcumol) and crystal I (curcuma zedoary) obtained from Wenyu gold oil, the test found that mouse sarcoma S37, cervix U14, and Ehrlich ascites carcinoma EAC were all injected at 75 mg/kg subcutaneously. There is a higher inhibition rate, but the effect of S180 is weak.

If the tumor shrinks significantly, there is a significant increase in fibrocytes around the tumor tissue, with a layer of lymphocytes, phagocytes surrounding the tumor cells, and other immune reactions.

The observation under an electron microscope: It was found that the tumor cells in the treatment group had obvious changes, mainly in the reduction of nucleoplasm ratio, nuclear appearance tended to be normal, and the number of chromatin, nucleoli and interchromatin particles decreased.

It can be considered that curcumol has an inhibitory effect on the nuclear metabolism of mouse sarcoma.

In vitro test results, curcumol and curcumone have obvious damaging effects on Ehrlich ascites cancer cells and can make them degenerate and necrotic.

Two transplantable tumors, TM755 and R615 strains of 615 pure mice were used as models for in vivo treatment experiments.

Intraperitoneal injection of zedoary turmeric oil 50mg/kg in mice has achieved significant effects, and its tumor inhibition rate is 35%-60%.

Zedoary oil has a radiosensitizing effect on lung adenoma (LA-795).

The b-elemene extracted from turmeric can significantly prolong the survival time of ascites carcinoma and ascites reticulocyte sarcoma AR S mice.

At a therapeutic dose, the number of bone marrow nucleated cells in peripheral leukocytes is not reduced, that is, there is no significant inhibition of hematopoietic function.

b-elemene, zedoary turmeric oil has a direct cytotoxic effect on leukemia L615 cells in vitro, and can cause tumor cell degeneration and necrosis.

b-elemene can directly cause degeneration and necrosis of tumor cells of the mouse breast cancer Ca761-86 cell line, and multiple injections of elemene into the tumor.

It has a strong killing effect on liver cancer cells cultured in vitro.

B-elemene was injected into the abdominal cavity of Ehrlich ascites cancer mice, and the morphology of the cancer cells was obviously changed under the microscope until the cells ruptured.

b-elemene is the Ehrlich ascites cancer cell with significantly less nucleic acid content, especially the reduction of RNA content is more significant.

The anti-cancer action of turmeric has direct effects and also involves the immune response of the host.

It has been observed clinically that zedoary turmeric oil tumors were injected into the body, and part of the cancer tissue was necrotic and shedding, and the cervix became smooth, achieving clinical treatment.

These morphological changes suggest that Zedoary has a direct cancer-killing effect.

In the pathological section, there are dense lymphocytes surrounding the cancer cells.

There are a large number of sinus cell tissues proliferating in Linpa sinus,

Lymphocytes in the blood after re-use of turmeric have a significant increase, etc.

All suggest that the host has an obvious immune response in effective cases.

18. Z-C-Q LBP
Anti-tumor ingredients:
Lycium burbarurn polysaceharides (LBP)
The structure:
The main components are arabinose, glucose,
galactose, mannose, xylose, rhamnose, etc.
The existing parts:

Extracted from the body of fruit or raised from the fruit.

Anti-tumor effect:

1. The experiments of Wang Baikun and other scholars proved:

    1) LBP has the effect of enhancing the cellular immune function of normal mice.

    2) At a dose of 10mg/kg, it can improve the cellular immune function of S180 tumor-bearing mice, and at the same time have anti-tumor effects.

    3) And it has a synergistic anti-tumor effect with the chemotherapeutic drug cyclophosphamide, especially when cyclophosphamide cy has no obvious anti-tumor effect.

2. There are also reports:

LBP has a certain influence on immune function.

Lv Changxing and others reported:

LBP combined with radiotherapy showed obvious radiosensitization.

3. In addition, the Betaine contained in its root bark also has anti-tumor effects.

4. Compatible with D-isoascorbic acid, it can inhibit the mitosis of sarcoma 37, Ehrlich's carcinoma and lymphoid leukemia L1210 in vitro, **and the effect is called single drug.**

5. The β-sitosterol and ascorbic acid contained in LBP have certain anti-tumor effects.

6. There are also reports:

LBP and interleukin-2 have a regulatory effect on the anti-tumor activity of two LAK cells in mice.

7. The experiments show that:

The tumor weight inhibition rate of Lycium barbarum on S180 solid tumor in mice was 42%.

Intraperitoneal injection of LBP 10mg/kgxd or 20mg/kg xd x7, the tumor inhibition rate on mouse S180 was 31% and 39%, respectively.

8. In vitro experiments it shows that:

Lycium barbarum has a significant inhibitory effect on human gastric adenocarcinoma LATP-L cells and human cervical cancer Hel a cells.

Its mechanism of action is mainly manifested in inhibiting cell DNA synthesis, interfering with cell division, and reducing the ability of cells to reproduce.

9. For observation of the ultrastructure of cancer cells it was to found that the changes to mitochondria were the most obvious.

19. XZ-C-R
Panax pseudo-Wall, var.notoginseng Hooet Tseng
Anti-tumor ingredients:
Panax Notoginsenoside R1; Notogiiisenoside R1
The effective parts:
It is the root of the plant.
Anti-tumor effect:

After treatment with notoginsenoside R180ug/ml for 5 days, 68% of HL-60 cells can be induced to differentiate, which proves that notoginsenoside R1 is a strong inducer of HL-60 cell line.

It can induce neutrophil differentiation of HL-60 cells.

The results of H-TdR incorporation experiments proved that notoginsenoside R1 can induce the differentiation of HL-60 cells, and at the same time affect the synthesis of cellular DNA and RNA.

It has also been reported that the anti-tumor activity of mouse splenocytes induced by notoginsenosides was studied by Cr release experiment, and it was found that the induced cells have strong anti-tumor effect in the presence of ConA/PHA.

Further experiments showed that Panax notoginseng saponins have no stimulating effect on the proliferation of spleen cells, but can change the content of CAMP in spleen cells.

20. Z-C-Z1
Coriololus versicolor Quel.
Anti-tumor ingredients:
Polysocohartibe-piptide
The structure:

There are many a, b (1-4) fucans as the main chain, the molecule contains about 15% of the protein, and there are 18 amino acids connected at the same time.

The existing parts:
The mycelium of this product
Anti-tumor effect:

Human gastric cancer cell line (S0C7901), human lung adenocarcinoma cell line (SPC), human monocytic leukemia cell line ((SLY), human skin tissue cell lymphoma cell line (MEl) were selected as target cells, and PSK was used for In vitro tumor inhibition test.

The results show that PS K has a moderate inhibitory effect on the proliferation of target cells, and can still cause a series of abnormal morphological changes on human lung adenocarcinoma cell lines (SPC) at a concentration of 1000ug/ml.

PSK (Kretsin) obtained by Japanese scholars is effective in sarcoma 180, liver cancer AH-13, AH-7974, AH-66F, and leukemia P388.

Intravenous, intraperitoneal, subcutaneous or oral administration is almost non-toxic, and its principle of action is believed to improve the immune function of the host through "host-mediated" action.

Scholars such as Yu Lijian reported:

Yunzhi extract has no obvious inhibitory effect on ascites liver cancer in mice transplanted subcutaneously, but on the 12th day after tumor transplantation, the extract showed obvious inhibitory effect on mouse ascites sarcoma S180 transplanted subcutaneously.

With time, the anti-tumor effect is greatly weakened.

Scholars such as Wang Supin reported:

The anti-tumor effect experiment was carried out on 5 kinds of Changbai Mountain Yunzhi polysaccharides with different structures,

The results show that this product has the effect of inhibiting the growth of liver cancer in mice and prolonging the survival period of liver cancer mice.

The different structural formulations of this product have different effects on the inhibition rate of liver cancer in mice and the life extension rate of mice, suggesting that the tumor inhibition rate is related to the polysaccharide structure, but its regularity is not clear.

Also reported:

The effect of Shaanxi Yunzhi extract on the macrophage activity of tumor-bearing mice was studied.

Ni Naile and other scholars reported on the morphological study of the anti-tumor effect of Shaanxi Yunzhi and Changbai Mountain Yunzhi extracts.

There are reports abroad:

The Yunzhi glycoprotein (PSK) extracted from Yunzhi and doxorubicin are used in tumor-bearing mice to inhibit tumor growth, improve the survival rate of mice and restore the transplanted immune function.

Doxorubicin alone can inhibit tumor growth, but the survival rate cannot be significantly improved due to side effects. Combined use of PSK and adriamycin can produce anti-tumor, low-toxicity synergistic effects.

Adriamycin has an inhibitory effect on the immune function of tumor-bearing mice, and PSK can restore the animal's immune function suppressed by doxorubicin. There are also research reports on the combination of PSK and mitomycin C. The combination of the two drugs (PO or ip) can delay the growth of tumors in mice, improve survival time, and restore suppressed immunity. The combined drug is more effective than the two drugs alone. Significant use.

The anti-tumor activity of Yunzhi polysaccharide fraction and its influence on immune function,

(Moon) CK and other scholars also conducted research:

It was found that copolang polysaccharide (copolang) and PSK showed almost the same anti-tumor activity, and significantly enhanced antibody-mediated allergic reactions in tumor mice, delayed hypersensitivity reactions and NK cell activity,

However, it has no effect on the function of antibody secreting cells and macrophages in normal mice.

It is suggested that the anti-tumor activity of Yunzhi polysaccharide can be compared with PSK.

In clinical use, Yunzhi intracellular polysaccharides are used to treat primary liver cancer. Single use can improve clinical symptoms and prolong life. Combined with anti-tumor drugs, it can also reduce the side effects of anti-tumor drugs.

Japan has developed proteoglycan "PSK" anti-cancer drugs.

21. Lentinus edodes Sing
Anti-tumor component A:
Lentinan
Structural formula:

Its structure is ß-D-(1 3) pyran glucan backbone.

Every five D-glucosyl C-6 has two fulcrums, connecting the branched chain composed of ß-D-(1 6) and ß-D-(1,3) glucose, which may also contain a small amount of 3- D-(1, 6) branched chain.

Existing part:
Its fruit body
Its anti-tumor effect:

Lentinan has a certain anti-tumor effect and improves the body's immunity.

At the dose of 0.2, 1, 5, 25 mg/kg, intraperitoneal injection every day for 10 consecutive days. After 5 weeks, the inhibition rate of sarcoma S180 was 78, 95.1, 97.5, 73%, respectively.

Compatibility with chemotherapeutics can enhance its anti-tumor effect.

Lentinai has a cytotoxic effect on human peripheral monocytes (PMNC are mainly lymphocytes) DNA synthesis, immunoglobulin and interferon induction, non-specific cell mediation.

It has an inhibitory effect on the number and proliferation of PMNC after chemotherapy.

It can enhance the cytotoxic response of natural killer cells (NK).

The vitality of NK cells in PMNC of leukemia patients is extremely low or even absent. Treatment with general immune enhancers may increase the risk of leukocyte canceration, while Lentinan can increase the vitality of NK cells.

The r-IFN induced by it has a stronger anti-cancer effect than a and ß-IFN.

And can enhance the patient's leukocyte phagocytic activity and opsonin production.

At the same time, it can also prevent the infection of tumor patients by bacteria and viruses.

Research by Shiio T et al shows:

Lentinan and chemotherapeutics have the inhibitory effect on lung metastasis of tumors in mice. Lentina is the most effective after postoperative administration.

Fachet T et al. found that Lentinan and its preparations have significant anti-tumor activity against A/ph, MC, S1 fibrosarcoma in A/ph and (A/ph B10) F1 hybrid mice. However, Lentinan does not directly affect tumor growth in vitro.

Shiio T et al also studied the inhibitory effect of Lentinan on lung metastasis of cancer.

Intravenous injection of Lentinan inhibits the metastasis of Lewis lung cancer (3 LL), melanoma (B6) and cellulosarcoma (ML-CS-1) in mice.

11

The exclusive development products of the scientific research: The series products of XZ-C immune regulation anti-cancer Chinese medicine

(introduction)

The self-developed XZ-C (XU ZE China) immunomodulatory anti-cancer series of traditional Chinese medicine preparations, from the experimental research to clinical verification, is applied to clinical practice based on the success of animal experiments. After years of clinical verification of a large number of clinical cases, the effect is remarkable. It is the independent invention achievements, the independent innovation and the independent intellectual property rights.

The research on searching and screening anti-cancer and anti-metastatic drugs from traditional Chinese medicine are the following processes:

1. *The purpose is to screen out new anti-cancer, anti-cancer, anti-metastatic and anti-relapse intelligent anti-cancer new drugs that have no drug resistance, no toxic and side effects, high selectivity and long-term oral administration.*

It is well known that the anticancer agents used in the world can indeed inhibit the proliferation of cancer cells, but it kills both cancer cells and normal cells, especially bone marrow immune cells, and seriously damages the host, because the chemotherapeutic cytotoxic agents are not selective. Moreover, traditional chemotherapy suppresses immune function and bone marrow hematopoietic function. Traditional intravenous chemotherapy is an intermittent treatment, which cannot be treated during the interstitial period, however, the cancer cells continue to proliferate and divide in the interstitial period.

Although chemotherapeutic drugs can inhibit the proliferation of cancer cells, it has to be stopped when the cancer has not completely been eliminated because of its toxic and side effects.

After stopping the drug, the cancer cells proliferated again and began to become resistant. When drug resistance occurs, this dose will not work, so it is to increase the dose. However, if the dose is increased, it may endanger the patient's life. If the given chemotherapeutic drug is resistant, it will not only have no effect on cancer cells, but will only kill the patient's normal cells. Therefore, the resistance of cancer cells to anticancer drugs and the side effects of anticancer drugs on the host are long-term troublesome problems.

Therefore, the purpose of the new drugs we are looking for is to avoid these shortcomings.

According to the theory of cell proliferation cycle, the anticancer agent must be used for a long time, so that the cancer focus can be continuously bathed in the anticancer agent for a long time, so as to stop its cell division and prevent recurrence and metastasis. It must be carried out over a long period of time, and it is best to take a long-term oral medicine to inhibit the existing cancer foci and prevent the formation of new cancer cells. The current anti-cancer drugs are not likely to be used for a long period of time due to the large toxic and side effects, but can only be used according to the treatment course and short cycle. Existing anticancer drugs all suppress immune function, suppress bone marrow hematopoiesis, suppress thymus, and suppress the side effects of bone marrow. ***The formation and development of cancer is due to the loss of immune function in the patient and the loss of immune surveillance. Therefore, all cancer drugs should increase immune function and protect immune organs, and should not use drugs that suppress immune function.***

To this end, our laboratory conducted the following experimental research on screening new anti-cancer and anti-metastatic drugs from traditional Chinese medicine.

1. The experiment as the following:

(1) *Using the method of cultivating cancer cells in vitro to conduct screening experimental research on the anti-tumor rate of Chinese herbal medicine*

In vitro screening test:

Use cancer cells in vitro to observe the direct damage of drugs to cancer cells.

In the test tube screening test, place raw and crude drugs (500ug / ml) in the test tubes of the cultured cancer cells to observe whether they have inhibitory effects on cancer cells or not.

We selected 200 kinds of Chinese herbal medicines that traditional Chinese medicine believes have anti-cancer effects, and conducted in vitro screening tests one by one.

And it was to culture with normal fibroblasts under the same conditions, to test the drug's toxicity to this cell, and then to compare.

(2) *Manufacture cancer-bearing animal models, and conduct an experimental screening study on the tumor suppressing rate of Chinese herbal medicines on cancer-bearing animals*

In vivo cancer suppression screening test, 240 mice in each batch were divided into 8 groups, 30 in each group, the 7th group was a blank control group, and the 8th group used 5-Fu or CTX as a control group.

All mice inoculated with EAC or S180 or H22 cancer cells.

After 24 hours of inoculation, each rat was orally fed raw and crude medicine powder, and the long-term feeding of the selected traditional Chinese medicine was conducted to monitor the survival time and toxicity, calculate prolonged survival rate, calculate cancer suppression rate.

In this way, we have carried out 4 years of the experimental research, and 3 years of experimental research on the pathogenesis, metastasis and recurrence mechanism of tumor-bearing mice, and experimental research <u>to explore how and why tumors cause host death.</u>

More than 1,000 tumor-bearing animal models are used every year, and a total of nearly 6000 tumor-bearing animal models have been made in 4 years.

After the death of each experimental rat, pathological anatomy of liver, spleen, lung, thymus, and kidney was performed, and a total of more than 20,000 slices <u>***were taken to explore whether there may be a small pathogen that causes cancer.***</u>

<u>***Microcirculation microscope was used to observe the establishment of tumor microvessels and microcirculation in 100 tumor-bearing mice***</u>.

Through experimental research, we have discovered for the first time in China that the traditional Chinese medicine TG has a significant effect on the inhibition of tumor microvessel formation. It has been used in clinical anti-metastatic treatment in more than 80 patients, and its efficacy is being observed.

2. The experimental results:

Among the 200 kinds of Chinese herbal medicines selected by animal experiments in our laboratory, 48 kinds are indeed selected, and they even have an excellent inhibitory effect on cancer cell proliferation. The tumor inhibition rate is above 75-90%.

However, there are some commonly used traditional Chinese medicines that are believed to have anti-cancer effects. After in vitro animal screening, in vivo tumor suppression rate screening has no effect or little effect. In this group, 152 species were eliminated by animal experiment screening without obvious anti-cancer effect.

The 48 flavored traditional Chinese medicines screened by this experiment did have a better cancer suppression rate, and then the optimized combination was repeated to carry out the cancer suppression rate experiment in vivo, and finally developed an immunomodulatory anti-cancer Chinese medicine with Chinese characteristics XU ZE China1 -10 preparation (XZ-C$_{1-10}$).

XZ-C1 can significantly inhibit cancer cells, but does not affect normal cells; Z-C4 can promote thymus hyperplasia and increase immunity; XZ-C8 can protect marrow and blood, and protect bone marrow hematopoiesis.

3. Clinical validation

Based on the success of animal experiments, it was to perform clinical verification.

That is to establish an outpatient center for cancer oncology and the collaboration group for anti-cancer, anti-metastasis, and recurrence research that combines Chinese and Western medicine, retain outpatient medical records, establish a regular follow-up observation system, and observe long-term efficacy.

It was from experimental research to clinical verification, new problems were discovered during the clinical verification process, and then returned to the laboratory for basic research, and then the new experimental results were applied to clinical verification.

So, it is the experiment-clinical-re-experiment-re-clinical, all experimental research must pass clinical verification.

It was the observation for 3-5 years in a large number of patients, and even the clinical observation is 8-10 years.

According to evidence-based medicine, there are long-term follow-up and evaluable data, and it was proved that it is clear that it has good long-term efficacy.

The standard of efficacy is:
Good quality of life and long life span

XZ-C immunomodulated anti-cancer traditional Chinese medicine has been tested by a large number of mid-to-late cancer patients, and has achieved remarkable results.

XZ-C immune-modulating anti-cancer Chinese medicine can improve the quality of life of patients with advanced cancer, enhance immunity, increase the body's ability to fight cancer, increase appetite, and significantly prolong survival.

The brief introduction is as follows:

(1). <u>**The study on the Mechanism of XZ-C Immunomodulatory Anticancer Chinese Medicine**</u>

With the continuous deepening of the research on traditional Chinese medicine, many traditional Chinese medicines are known to have a regulatory effect on the production and biological activity of cytokines and other immune molecules.

At this time, the immunological mechanism of XZ-C immune regulation and control anti-cancer traditional Chinese medicine elucidated at the molecular level has significantly important meaning.

1). XZ-C anti-cancer Chinese medicine can protect immune organs and increase the weight of thymus and spleen.

2). XZ-C anti-cancer Chinese medicine has obvious promotion effect on bone marrow cell proliferation and hematopoietic function.

3). XZ-C anti-cancer Chinese medicine can enhance the immune function of T cells, and obviously promote the proliferation of T cells.

4). XZ-C anti-cancer Chinese medicine has a significant enhancement effect on the production of human IL-2.

5). XZ-C anti-cancer traditional Chinese medicine has activation and enhancement effects on NK cell activity.

NK cells have a broad-spectrum anti-tumor effect and can kill heterogeneous tumor cells.

6). XZ-C anti-cancer Chinese medicine can enhance the activity of LAK cells.

LAK cells can kill solid tumor cells sensitive and insensitive to NK cells, and have a broad-spectrum anti-tumor effect.

7). XZ-C anti-cancer Chinese medicine has an inducing effect and an promoting inducing-effect on interferon (INF).

    a. *IFN has a broad-spectrum anti-tumor effect and immunoregulatory effect.*

    b. *IFN can inhibit the proliferation of tumor cells.*

    c. *IFN can activate NK cells and CTL to kill tumors cell.*

8). XZ-C anti-cancer traditional Chinese medicine has the effect of enhancing the colony stimulating factor.

CSF not only participates in the proliferation and differentiation of hematopoietic cells, but also plays an important role in the host's tumor immunity.

9). XZ-C anti-cancer Chinese medicine can promote tumor necrosis factor (TNF).

TNF is a type of cytokine that can directly cause tumor cell death. Its main biological role is to kill or inhibit tumor cells.

    (2). Biological response modifiers (BRM) and BRM-like traditional Chinese medicine and tumor treatment

1. Biological response modifiers (BRM) have opened up new areas of tumor biotherapy. At present, BRM, as the fourth type of tumor therapy, has received extensive attention from the medical community.

In 1982, Oldham founded the biological response modifier (BRM), or BRM theory.

On this basis, the family proposed the fourth modality of cancer treatment (four modality of cancer treatment)-biological treatment in 1984.

__According to the BRM theory__, under normal circumstances, the tumor and the body's defense are in a dynamic balance. The occurrence of tumors and even invasion and metastasis are completely or entirely caused by the imbalance of this dynamic balance. If the disordered state is artificially adjusted to a normal level, the growth of the tumor can be suppressed and resolved. In other words, if the already disordered state is artificially adjusted to a normal level, the growth of the tumor can be controlled and it can be regressed.

Specifically, BRM includes the following anti-tumor mechanisms:

1) *It is to promote the enhancement of the host defense mechanism effect, or reduce the immune suppression of the tumor-bearing host, so as to achieve the immune response to the cancer.*

2) *It is to inject natural or genetically reorganized biologically active substances to enhance the host's defense mechanism.*

3) *It is to modify tumor cells to induce a strong host response.*

4) *It is to promote the differentiation and maturation of tumor cells and normalize them.*

5) *It is to reduce the side effects of cancer chemotherapy and radiotherapy, and enhance the tolerance of the host.*

2. BRM-like effect and curative effect of XZ-C immune regulation and control anti-cancer traditional Chinese medicine:

XZ-C immunomodulated anti-cancer Chinese medicine has been shown to have BRM-like effects and therapeutic effects after 4 years of experimental studies on cancer-bearing animals and 40 years of clinical verification. It is a BRM-like drug that has been screened and discovered from Chinese medicine resources.

XZ-C immunomodulated anti-cancer Chinese medicine was screened out of 200 Chinese herbal medicines by Professor Xu Ze's laboratory. First, the cancer cells were cultured in vitro, and 200 kinds of Chinese herbal medicines were screened in vitro one by one to observe the experimental research on the direct damage of each medicine to the cancer cells in the culture tube. And the comparison test of tumor inhibition rate with the chemotherapy drug CTX and normal cells cultured in test tube as the control group. As a result, a batch of drugs that have a certain inhibitory rate on cancer cell proliferation were selected. And then it was further to create tumor-bearing animal models and conduct experimental screening research on the in vivo tumor inhibition rate of tumor-bearing animal models on 200 Chinese herbal medicines. For each medication, the scientific, objective and rigorous experimental screening, analysis, and evaluation are carried out on a taste of medication by a taste of medication.

In the end, the experiments have shown that only 48 kinds of tumors do have a good tumor suppression rate, while another 152 commonly used Chinese herbal medicines have been screened by the tumor suppression rate of this group of tumor-bearing experiments, which proves that there is no anti-cancer effect or the tumor suppression rate is very small.

The XZ-C immune regulation and control anti-cancer metastatic Chinese medicines that have indeed a good tumor suppression rate were selected through the above experiments.

It has the functions of improving immunity, increasing thymus weight, protecting thymus tissue, improving cellular immunity, promoting bone marrow cell proliferation, protecting bone marrow hematopoiesis, increasing the number of red blood cells and white blood cells, enhancing cell function, activating immune cytokines, and improving the immune monitoring function in blood flow.

The main pharmacological effect of XZ-C immunomodulatory anti-cancer Chinese medicine is anti-cancer and increasing immunity, and its anti-cancer mechanism is:

1). It is to activate the body's immune cell system, promote the enhancement of host defense mechanism effects, and achieve the immune response to cancer.

2). It is to activate the immune cytokine system of the body's anti-cancer mechanism, enhance the host defense mechanism and improve the immune surveillance of the immune cells of the body's blood circulation system.

3). It is to protect the thymus gland, protect the thymus gland, increase immunity, protect the marrow and generate blood, protect the bone marrow and hematopoietic function, stimulate the bone marrow hematopoietic function, promote the recovery of the bone marrow system, increase white blood cells, red blood cells, etc.

4). It is to reduce the side effects of radiotherapy and chemotherapy, and enhance the host's tolerance.

5). It can increase the weight of the thymus and prevent the thymus from progressive atrophy, because the thoracic atrophy is progressive when the cancer progresses.

As mentioned above, the mechanism of action of XZ-C immunomodulatory anti-cancer traditional Chinese medicine is basically similar to that of BRM, and its clinical treatment also obtains the same therapeutic effect as BRM. Or in another word, it has the same therapeutic effect of BRM can be obtained in clinical use.

Therefore, XZ-C immunomodulatory anti-cancer Chinese medicine has BRM-like effects and curative effects. It combines the current advanced molecular oncology theory with ancient Chinese herbal medicine resources at the molecular level and it uses BRM theory as a bridge to integrate with the advanced theories and practices of international modern molecular oncology.

(One)

XZ-C1 "Intelligent Suppression of Cancer"

1.【Main Ingredients】

Eight anti-cancer medicines such as Longya grass and Shuyangquan, etc

2. Anticancer pharmacology

1). Clearing away heat and detoxifying, promoting blood circulation and removing blood stasis, supporting the body and strengthening the essential or root of the body, removing evil without hurting the right, strongly inhibiting cancer cells, inhibiting cancer cell metastasis, and not inhibiting normal cells.

2). It has inhibitory activity on mouse Ehrlich ascites cancer cells in anti-cancer test in mice. There is a significant difference between the administration group and the control group.

3). It can prolong the survival time of cancer-bearing mice and improve the survival rate of mice by 26. 92%.

4). The main drugs XZ-C1-A, XZ-C1-B in the prescription have a stable and significant anticancer effect, 100% inhibition of cancer cells; in the administration group cancer cells have reduced mitotic phases, and degeneration and necrosis are serious. It has no effect on epithelial cells or fiber cells.

The water extract of XZ-C1-D in the prescription has inhibitory activity on human uterine cancer cells, and the inhibition rate of mouse sarcoma S180 is as high as 98.9%.

Other flavors in the prescription also have strong anti-cancer effects.

5). The anti-tumor effect of XZ-C1 Chinese medicine on H22 mice bearing liver cancer:

The tumor inhibition rate of XZ-C1 was 40% in the second week, 45% in the fourth week, and 58% in the sixth week.

In the control group with CTX medication, the tumor inhibition rate was 45% in the second week, 45% in the fourth week, and 49% in the sixth week.

6). The effect of XZ-C1 traditional Chinese medicine on the survival time of H22-bearing mice:

The life extension rate of the XZ-C1 group was 85%, and the life extension rate of the CTX control group (chemotherapy drug cyclophosphamide) was 9.8%.

3. Clinical application

1). The indications:

Esophageal cancer, gastric cancer, colorectal cancer, lung cancer, breast cancer, liver cancer, bile duct cancer, pancreatic cancer, thyroid cancer, nasopharyngeal cancer, brain tumor, kidney cancer, bladder cancer, ovarian cancer, cervical cancer, various sarcomas, and various metastatic and recurrent cancer.

2). The usage:

After XZ-C1 was served for 1-3 months continueously, the patients felt effective about themselves, and it can be taken for a long time.

It can be taken every other day after three years and 2 times per week after 5 years so that it can keep immune function and cytokines maintain at a certain level for a long period, that is, the immune function and cytokines can be maintained at a certain level for a long time.

4.Toxicity test

a. XZ-C1 can be taken long.

b. The acute toxicity experiment showed that when the mice were gavaged at 10 times of the adult dose (10g / Kg body weight) and observed at 24, 48, 72, and 96 hours, none of the 30 purebred mice died.

c. The half lethal dose (LD50) is difficult to make and is a fairly safe prescription.

d. It has been used in this oncology clinic for many years. Some patients in the clinic have been taking it for 3-5 years for a long time, and may also take it for 8-10 years to maintain the body's immunity and prevent recurrence and metastasis.

e. This prescription can be taken for a long time and is quite a safe oral anticancer drug.

(Two)

XZ-C2
Anticancer pharmacology

1. Animal experiments can prolong the survival time of L7211 mice (leukemia mice). Compared with the control group, it has significant statistical significance.

2. It can increase the inhibition rate of L7211 mice.

3. XZ-C1-A and XZ-C1-B have a strong inhibitory effect on mouse sarcoma (S180).

The **Clinical application**

a. The Indications:

1. Leukemia, upper gastrointestinal cancer, tongue cancer, laryngeal cancer, nasopharyngeal cancer, esophageal cancer, cervical cancer, bone metastasis. Esophageal or gastric cancer recurrent stenosis after anastomosis (cannot be re-operated).

2. It is general effect on acute lymphocytic leukemia, but it has a significant effect on other types of leukemia;

3. It has a significant effect on the inhibition of bone metastasis.

b. The usage:

Generally, 1 capsule Qid or 2 capsules tid

Leukemia 3 capsules after tid meal, 7 days as a course of treatment.

(Three)

XZ-C3
Cancer pain-free powder and application for external acupoint
Anticancer pharmacology

1. It is to clean away heat and detoxifying, diminish inflammation and relieve pain, relieve qi and dissipating pain;

2. It promotes blood circulation, removes blood stasis, reduces swelling and relieves pain, plays a role in clearing away heat and detoxification, reducing swelling and analgesic effects, and among all of the above, the analgesic effects are most prominent.

3. It is suitable for acupuncture point effect stickers, which can better exert the drug effect and achieve the purpose of rapid pain relief than simply applying the pain.

The prescription content
The basic recipe: 14 flavors such as shanna and turmeric, etc
Clinical application

a. Indications:

Liver cancer; lung cancer pain; pancreatic cancer back pain; bone cancer pain points; neck and, or supraclavicular metastatic lymph node mass.

b. The usage:

It is to be ground into details. Take an appropriate amount of honey, mix and stir evenly into a paste for later use, to form a paste. d

For the lung cancer, to apply to Rugen point (5th and 6th intercostal space under the nipple), and liver cancer to apply to Jimen point (6-7 intercostal space on the midline of breast). For lung cancer, apply to Rugen (the 5th and 6th intercostal nipple straight down).

Liver cancer is applied to the Qimen acupoint (between the 6-7 intercostals of the breast line),

After applying the medicine, cover it with gauze track and fix it with tape.

If the pain is severe, it will be changed once every 6 hours.

For those with lighter or mild pain, replace it once every 12 hours and continue to use it until the pain eases or disappears. Or use it continuously until the pain is relieved or disappears.

The experience for this medication:

It is used to treat 84 cases of the patients with liver cancer and pneumonia pain. They all have analgesic effects. Generally, 3 times of medication treatment can relieve the pain to different degrees, or usually with 3 times of medication, the pain can be reduced to varying degrees. After 3-7 days, they have obvious analgesic effects or there is obvious analgesic effect, and some have basic analgesics, or some are basically analgesic, or the patient's pain stop.

(Four)

XZ-C4
Protection of Thymus and Increase immune function
or Cancer-Free Medication (5g/ bag)

1. [Main ingredients]
12 valuable Chinese herbal medicines such as ginseng and ganoderma
2. Anticancer pharmacology

1. Promote the transformation of lymphocytes, enhance the anti-cancer cellular immune function, increase white blood cells, inhibit cancer cells, and warm up qi and blood.

2. Ehrlich ascites cancer cells were transplanted into the abdominal cavity of mice. The mice were given chemotherapy drugs twice on the first day and the seventh day after transplantation. At the same time, taking XZ-C4 (2g / kg) every day significantly enhanced the efficacy of chemotherapy drugs effect.

3. When MMC is used for chemotherapy, it can inhibit the leukopenia and weight loss caused by MMC.

4. Anticancer chemical drugs were injected into the veins of cancer bearing mice while taking XZ-C4. It was found that the effect of inhibiting cancer cells was three times higher than that of chemotherapy drugs alone.

5. The chemotherapeutic drugs damage the thymus, spleen and other immune organs of cancer-bearing mice, but after taking XZ-C4, the thymus, spleen and other organs do not shrink completely, indicating that XZ-C4 immune organs play a protective role.

6. After giving the XZ-C4 extract of Ehrlich ascites carcinoma mice, the life extension rate of the mice was as high as 167.1%; the survival time of the control group mice was 15.2 days on average, while the XZ-C4 administration group was 25.4 days. Meanwhile, it shows that the function of mouse reticuloendothelial system is obviously high.

7. XZ-C4 can quickly reduce the side effects of the chemotherapeutic agent cisplatin, and can improve the efficacy of cisplatin. XZ-C4 can inhibit the toxic and side

effects of cisplatin 100%, and the dosage is just the normal daily amount of humans. Or, the dosage is the daily routine amount of a person.

XZ-C4 does not resist the cancer resistance of cisplatin. XZ-C4 can protect the kidneys, so that renal damage of cisplatin hardly occurs.

XZ-C4 is a clinically promising anti-cancer powder.

8. The use of XZ-C4 has a significant effect on patients after cancer surgery. After radical surgery for gastrointestinal, hepatopancreas and other cancers, they all show physical strength, immunity, fatigue, anorexia, and anemia.

Within 1-2 weeks after the operation, starting from being able to take oral or gastric tube feeding, taking XZ-C granules orally, 7.5 grams per day, taking 3 times before meals, the course of treatment is 12 weeks, during this time period which chemotherapy or immunotherapy can be performed.

9. Anti-tumor effect of XZ-C4 traditional Chinese medicine on H_{22} mice bearing liver cancer:

The XZ-C4 medication had a tumor inhibition rate of 55% at the second week, 68% at the fourth week, and 70% at the sixth week, and in the CTX (cyclophosphamide) control group at the second week the tumor inhibition rate was 45%, and the disease suppression rate at week 4 was 49%.

10. The effect of XZ-C4 traditional Chinese medicine on the survival time of H_{22} mice bearing liver cancer:

The survival rate of XZ-C4 group was 200%, and that of CTX group was 9.8%.

11. XZ-C4 can significantly improve immune function, increase white blood cells and red blood cells, has no effect on liver and kidney functions, and does not damage liver and kidney slices. CTX reduces leukocytes, lowers immune function, and kidney slices have kidney damage.

12. The thymus in XZ-C4 treatment group is not atrophy and slightly hypertrophy, the thymus in CTX control group is obviously atrophy. XZ-C4 has a strong inhibitory effect on mouse sarcoma (S_{180}).

3. Clinical application

1). Indications:

a. Various cancers, sarcomas, various advanced cancers, metastases, recurrent cancers, adjuvant radiotherapy, chemotherapy, patients after surgery.

b. All kinds can be applied, especially dizziness, fatigue, tiresome or weakness, laziness, low energy, spontaneous sweating, palpitations, insomnia, qi and blood deficiency are more suitable.

c. It starts to take XZ-C immunomodulates anti-cancer traditional Chinese medicine before and after surgery.

It is to do clinical and laboratory tests every 4 weeks for 20 weeks.

The checked items are the following as:

The conscious and objective symptoms, body weight, total protein and albumin, total cholesterol, dielectric, ALT, AST blood routine and platelets, lymphocyte count, T cells and B cells, globulin, urine protein.

2). The treatment results:

① The number of lymphocytes has increased, and it has the effect of inhibiting leukopenia;

② No effect on liver function;

③ It has the function of protecting the kidneys, so as not to damage the kidneys;

④ It can significantly reduce the rash and stomatitis caused by chemotherapy and radiotherapy;

⑤ It is effective to restore physical strength after surgery, after chemotherapy, and after radiotherapy. It can increase appetite, improve overall burnout, and increase body weight.

XZ-C reduces the side effects of radiotherapy and chemotherapy, and improves the overall condition of the postoperative patient. It is a rare medicine for rehabilitation. Or It is a rare healing medicine.

The Experience from this medication as the following is:

Modern medicine has proposed a variety of treatments for advanced cancer, but there are still some problems. At present, it is not yet certain whether the combination of chemotherapy drugs or the combined use of chemotherapeutics for advanced cancer will be effective. Even if it is effective, it also brings serious toxic and side effects.

It can be considered that the treatment of cancer in modern medicine is to kill cancer cells and is aggressive, while traditional Chinese medicine controls and even eliminates cancer by enhancing the body's own adjustment function. Or, chinese medicine, on the other hand, enhances the body's own regulatory functions to control and even eliminate cancer.

To this end, it should find a treatment that reduces or eliminates symptoms, improves or treats the disease, has fewer side effects, and can prolong life. And XZ-C has such characteristics and advantages.

1). *XZ-C4 has the effect of enhancing the effect of anticancer drugs through experiments;*

2). *It has the effect of promoting the mitosis of B cells; it has the effect of promoting the recovery of radiation-damaged hematopoietic system;*

3). *it has the effect of promoting phagocytic cells;*

4). *It protects the thymus, improves immunity, and protects bone marrow to produce blood.*

2. Toxicity test

XZ-C4 can be taken for a long time.

Acute toxicity experiments have shown that the lethal dose (LD5O) cannot be achieved or cannot be tested and is a safe prescription.

It has been used for many years in this specialist clinic. Some patients have been taking it for 3-5 years or even 8-10 years to maintain the body's immunity and prevent cancer recurrence and metastasis. This prescription can be taken orally for a long time, it is quite safe anti-cancer and anti-metastatic oral drugs.

(Five)

The series preparations of the following XZ-C immune regulation and control anti-cancer Chinese medicine have many experimental and clinical contents and are long in length. Therefore, only the names are listed here, and the introduction is omitted.

1. XZ-C5 called as liver cancer powder is for liver cancer patient.

2. XZ-C6 called as bladder cancer powder is for the bladder cancer patient.

3. XZ-C7 called as lung cancer powder is for the lung cancer patient.

4. XZ-C8 is the medication which is used to protect the marrow and produce blood, and to attenuate the side effects caused by radiotherapy and chemotherapy.

5. XZ-C9 is the medication powder to be used for pancreatic cancer, prostate cancer.

6. XZ-C10 is called as Brain tumor powder which is used for brain cancer patient.

The above-mentioned scientific research Chinese medicine preparations for anti-cancer, anti-metastasis, and recurrence of various cancers, have been basically applied in clinical oncology specialist outpatient clinics for many years, and achieved good results.

The medication preparations from scientific research for treating various complications of cancer in our Oncology Clinic:

1). Kangxiaoshui Decoction-----Indications of pleural fluid and ascites

2). Shugan Jianghuang Decoction-----Indications of liver cirrhosis and jaundice

3). Postoperative Aikang San-----Helping recovery after radical cancer surgery

4). Hunger soup-----for cancer patients who have poor appetite

5). Tongyou Decoction-----for the cancer patient with postoperative anastomosed stenosis

6). Nianlian Songjie Decoction-----for patients with adhesions after cancer surgery

The above-mentioned preparations of scientific research Chinese medicine products, after many years of application observation in the outpatient department of this cancer specialist, all achieved good results, alleviated the suffering of patients, improved the quality of life, and prolonged the survival period.

Table The summary table of the main pharmacological effects of Z-C immune regulation anticancer Chinese herbal medicine (anti-cancer and increasing immune)

	Increased white blood cells	Enhanced phagocytosis	Enhance cellular immune	Enhance humoral immune	Enhanced hematopoietic function	Improve gastrointestinal function	Enhance the weight of the thymus	Promote bone marrow cell proliferation	Enhanced T cell function	Enhanced NK cell activity	Enhanced LAK cell activity	Enhanced IL-2 activity levels	Enhance the level of interferon IFN activity	Enhanced TNF activity levels	Enhanced CSF colony stimulating factor	Antagonistic WCBYC↓	Inhibition of platelet coagulation and antithrombosis	Antitumor	Anti-metastasis	Antiviral	Anti-cirrhosis	Liver protection	Eliminate free radicals	Protein synthesis	Anti-HIV	
Z-C-A-APL																		+	+							
Z-C-B-SLT																		+	+							
Z-C-C-SNL																		+	+							
Z-C-D-PGS	+	+	+	+	+	+	6	+	+	+	+	+	+	+	+	+	9	+	+	+			+	+		20
Z-C-E-PCW		+	+				2	+	+			+	+	+	+	+	7	+	+	+						12
Z-C-F-AMK		+	+	+	+	+	5			+			+			+	3	+		+		+				11
Z-C-G-GUF		+	+	+		+	4				+		+			+	3	+		+		+		+		11
Z-C-H-RGL	+		+		+		3		+	+			+	+		+	5	+					+			10
Z-C-I-PLP	+	+	+	+	+	+	6		+	+						+	3	+		+					+	12
Z-C-J-ASD	+	+	+	+	+		5	+	+	+			+	+	+	+	8	+				+				15
Z-C-K LWF		+	+				2						+			+	2	+	+							5
Z-C-L-AMB	+	+	+	+	+		5	+		+	+	+	+	+	+		7	+		+				+		5
Z-C-M LLA	+	+	+	+			4	+		+							2	+						+		5
Z-C-N-CZR		+					1						+			+	2	+	+							5
Z-C-O-PMT	+	+	+	+	+	+	6	+	+	+					+		4	+		+	+	+	+	+		16
Z-C-P-STG							0										0	+								1
Z-C-Q-LBP	+	+	+	+	+		5		+	+	+	+		+	+	+	8	+	+				4			16
Z-C-R-NSR		+					1	+			+					+	3	+	+		+	+				8
Z-C-S-GLK	+	+	+	+	+		5		+		+	+	+	+		+	6	+	+			+		+	+	16
Z-C-T-EDM	+	+	+	+	+		5	+		+			+	+	+	+	6	+		+			+			14
Z-C-U-PUF		+	+	+			3		+	+	+						3	+				+				8
Z-C-V-ABB							1		+	+	+			+			4	+								6

Z-C-W-SCB	+					1		+						+	2	+				+	+		5
Z-C-X-SDS						0			+	+	+				3	+					4
Z-C-Y-PAR						0			+	+	+		+	+	5	+				6
Z-C-Z-CVQ						0					+				1	+				2

XZ-C1 + XZ-C4 immunomodulating anti-cancer traditional Chinese medicine or XZ-C1+XZ-C4 immune regulation and control anti-cancer Chinese medicine

1. *It is to comprehensively improve the quality of life of advanced cancer patients.*

2. *It is to protect Thymus and to increase immune function, it is to protect marrow and produce blood, and it is to enhance immune function and to regulate and to control the immune function.*

3. *It is to enhance physical fitness and to relief pain and to increase appetite.*

4. *It is to enhance the treatment effect and reduce the side effects of chemotherapy.*

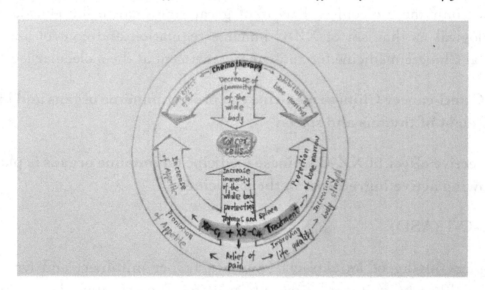

12

Research on the mechanism of XZ-C immune regulation and control of anti-cancer traditional Chinese medication

With the continuous in-depth study of Chinese medicine, it is known that many Chinese medicines can regulate the production and biological activities of cytokines and other immune molecules. This is of great significance for elucidating the immunological mechanism of XZ-C immune regulation and control anti-cancer traditional Chinese medicine for anti-cancer treatment at the molecular level.

1. **XZ-C anti-cancer Chinese medicine can protect immune organs and increase the weight of thymus and spleen**

The protective effect of XZ-C Chinese medicine on immune organs is played by the following active ingredients in the medicine:

1) **Z-C-T (ASD)**

Use 15g/kg, 30g/kg of its extracts (equal to 1g per milliliter) and ferulic acid suspension 12.5mg/kg, 25mg/kg daily to mice for 7 consecutive days, which can significantly increase mice Thymus and spleen weight. Especially in the high-dose group, the effect is more obvious.

Injecting its polysaccharide into the mice's abdominal cavity or Intraperitoneal injection of polysaccharides in mice can also significantly reduce the atrophy of the thymus and spleen caused by prednisolone.

2) Z-C-O(PMT)

The extract PM-2 was administered to normal mice with PMT 6g/(kg·d) decoction for 7 days, which can significantly increase the weight of the thymus and abdominal lymph nodes of the mice, and can antagonize the immunity caused by prednisolone The organ weight drops.

Giving 15-month-old mice its decoction (concentration of 0.5g/ml) 6g/kg for 14 days can significantly increase the weight and volume of the mouse thymus, thicken the cortex, and increase the cell density.

The combination of PM and Astragalus can significantly promote the proliferation of non-lymphocytes and ***help improve the microenvironment of the thymus.***

3) Z-C-W(SCB)

The polysaccharides of SCB can increase the weight of the thymus and spleen of normal mice.

Gavage with it can also increase the weight of the thymus and spleen of cyclophosphamide immunosuppressive mice.

4) Z-C-M(LLA)

Infusion of LLA decoction to mice for 7 days can significantly increase the weight index of mouse thymus and spleen.

5) Z-C-L

The thymus of 15-month-old mice degenerates significantly. Astragalus can significantly increase the thymus. Under light microscope, the cortex thickens and the cell density increases.

2. **The effect of XZ-C anti-cancer Chinese medicine on the proliferation, differentiation and hematopoietic function of bone marrow cells**

The following active ingredients of XZ-C Chinese medicine have an effect on bone marrow hematopoietic function as the following:

1). **XZ-C-Q (PMT) extract (PM-2) and Z-C-Q (LBP)**

a. The effect on normal mouse bone marrow hematopoietic stem cell proliferation (CFU-S):

Inject human PM-2 into experimental mice intravenously, at a dose of 50mg/(kgxd) X3d or LBP, at a dose of 10mg/(kg·d)X3d, and kill the test mice alive on the 9th day.

It was found that the number of CFU-S in the spleen of the mice in the administration group was significantly higher. The CFU-S of the PM-2 group and the LBP group were 121% and 136% of the control group, respectively.

b. The effect on normal mouse bone marrow macrophage colony forming unit (colony forming unit of granulooytes and macrophages, CFU-GM):

The experimental results show that LBP[5-3Omg/(kg·d)X3d] can significantly increase the number of CFU-GM, PM-2 can also significantly enhance the effect of CFU-GM, the effective dose is 12.5-50mg/(kg●d) X3d, CFU-GM is dominated by granulocyte colonies in the early stage of culture, then the macrophage colonies gradually increase, and the macrophage colonies dominate in the later period.

It can be seen from the above experiments that PM-2 and LBP have a significant promotion effect on the hematopoietic function of normal mice.

c. Experimental proof:

During the recovery process of cyclophosphamide-induced hematopoietic damage in mice, PM-2 and LEP first stimulated the proliferation of granule progenitor cells, and then the bone marrow nucleation promoted the increase, and finally showed to promote the recovery of the number of peripheral granulocytes.

2). XZ-C-D (TSPG) total ginsenosides are:

1)). The effective ingredients of ginseng to promote hematopoietic function,

2)). It can promote the recovery of peripheral red blood cells, hemoglobin and femoral bone marrow suppressor cells in myelosuppressive mice,

3)). Improve the division index of bone marrow cells,

4)). Stimulate the proliferation of bone marrow hematopoietic cells in vitro to enter the active cell cycle (S+ G2/M phase).

5)). TSPG can promote the proliferation and differentiation of pluripotent hematopoietic stem cells (CFU-S) and myeloid hematopoietic progenitor cells.

6)). TSPG can induce the production of hematopoietic growth factor (HGF).

3). XZ-C-H (RGL) Rehmannia glutinosa

1)). It can promote the recovery of red blood cells and hemoglobin in blood-deficient animals,

2)). Accelerate the proliferation and differentiation of bone marrow hematopoietic stem cells (CFU-S),

3)). It has a significant blood-producing effect.

4)). Continuous intraperitoneal injection of Rehmannia glutinosa polysaccharides into mice for 6 days can significantly promote the proliferation and differentiation of mouse bone marrow hematopoietic stem cells and progenitor cells.

5)). And increase the number of white blood cells in peripheral blood.

4). XZ-C-J (ASD) polysaccharide

a. It has no obvious effect on the red blood cells and hemoglobin of normal mice.

b. However, injection of ASD polysaccharides into mice showed significant effects on the proliferation and differentiation of multipotent hematopoietic stem cells (CFU-S) and hematopoietic progenitor cells of various lines of mice damaged by radiation.

c. But the decoction has no obvious effect.

5). XZ-C-E (PEW) Yunlingsu

a. (Small molecule compounds extracted from Yunling polysaccharide)

b. The effective part can enhance the production of colony stimulating factor (CSF) and increase the level of peripheral blood white blood cells in mice.

c. It can prevent the decrease of white blood cell level caused by cyclophosphamide, accelerate the recovery speed, and the effect is stronger than that of the white blood cell agent sodium ferulate.

6). XZ-C-Y (PAR)

a. Its polysaccharides can obviously resist the white blood cell reduction effect of cyclophosphamide,

b. Increase the number of bone marrow cells,

c. Promote CSF retention to induce bone marrow cell proliferation,

d. to promote the recovery and reconstruction of hematopoietic function of X-ray irradiated mice,

e. increase hematopoietic stem cells,

f. increase the number of bone marrow cells,

g. elevated white blood cells.

3. **XZ-C anti-cancer Chinese medicine can enhance the immune function of T cells**

The active or effective ingredients and functions of XZ-C Chinese medicine are as follows:

(1) Z-C-L (LBP)

a. it can significantly increase the percentage of peripheral blood lymphocytes in mice.

b. A small dose of LBP (5-10mg/kg) can cause lymphocyte proliferation, indicating that LBP has a significant effect on T cell proliferation.

c. Take 50mg/ (kgX d) x 7d as the optimal dose. Below this dose, there is no obvious promotion effect, and the effect will decrease if the dose exceeds this dose.

d. Oral LBP can increase the lymphocyte transformation rate of tumor patients with weak physical fitness and low white blood cells.

(2) XZ-C4

a. It has the function of regulating the immune system,

b. Can activate T cells in the collective lymph nodes,

c. Stimulate the secretion of hematopoietic growth factors in T cells.

d. Among the crude drugs that make up XZ-C4, the hot water extract of rhizome of Atractylodes lanceolata has obvious effect of stimulating lymph node cells, *which is considered to be the basis of XZ-C4 immune regulation.*

4. **XZ-C anti-cancer Chinese medicine activates and enhances NK cell activity**

a. Natural killer cells (NK cells) are another type of killer cells in human and mouse lymphocytes.

b. It can kill certain cells without antigen stimulation or antibody involvement.

c. It has an important immune function.

d. Especially in the body's immune surveillance function, NK cells are the first line of defense against tumors, and they have a relatively broad anti-tumor spectrum.

e. NK cells have a broad-spectrum anti-tumor effect, which can kill tumor cells of the same line, the same species and heterogeneity, especially for lymphoma and leukemia cells.

f. NK cells are an important type of immune regulatory cells,

g. It has a regulatory effect on T cells, B cells, bone marrow stem cells, etc., and regulates the body's immune function by releasing cytokines (such as IFN-a, IFN-y, IL-2, TNF, etc.).

The specific active ingredients and functions of XZ-C Chinese medicine are as follows:

1. **XZ-C-X Windproof (SDS)**

a. It can enhance the activity of NK cells in experimental mice.

b. When combined with IL-2, NK activity is higher.

c. It shows that Fangfeng polysaccharide promotes the activation of NK cells by IL-2 and helps to improve the activity of NK cells.

d. LBP can enhance T cell-mediated immune response and NK cell activity in normal mice and cyclophosphamide-treated mice.

e. Intraperitoneal injection of LBP can improve the proliferation of mouse spleen T lymphocytes and enhance the killing function of CTL.

The specific kill rate increased from 33% to 67%.

2. Z-C--G Glycyrrhizin (CL)

a. While inducing IFN in animal and human blood, it also enhances NK activity,

b. Clinical experiments by Abe et al. showed that intravenous injection of 80 mg of CL increased the cell activity by 75% in 21 patients, and intraperitoneal injection of 0.5 mg/kg GL in mice could enhance the activity of NK cells in the liver.

3. Z-C-L (AMB) liquid

a. It can significantly promote the activity of mouse NK cells in vivo and in vitro;

b. It can also directly induce mouse IFN-r when (AMB) is treated with effector cells at a certain concentration (0.1 l/mI),

c. Cordyceps alcohol extraction can enhance the activity of mouse NK cells in vivo and in vitro, and can significantly increase the activity of NK cells.

d. 0.5g/kg, 1g/kg, 5g/kg can significantly enhance mouse NK cell activity.

5. The effect of XZ-C anti-cancer Chinese medicine on lymphokine activated killer cells (LAK cell) activity

a. Lymphokine activated killer cells (LAK cells) can be induced by IL-2 cytokines.

b. LAK cells can kill solid tumor cells that are sensitive and insensitive to NK cells, and have a broad-spectrum anti-tumor effect.

c. XZ-C anti-cancer Chinese medicine specific active ingredients and functions:

(1). Z-C-L AMB polysaccharide

It can enhance the activity of LAK cells within a certain dose range, and 0.01mg/mi has the strongest effect, which is 3 times the killing effect of original LAK cells.

If its concentration is too high or too low, it has no effect.

(2). Z-C-U

It can significantly enhance the activity of spleen LAK cells in tumor-bearing mice to kill tumor cells and increase the activity of red blood cell C3b liquid.

PUPS and IL-2 have a synergistic effect, and can be used as a biological response modifier BRM for LAK/rIL-2 based tumor biological therapy.

(3). Z-C-V ABB polysaccharide

It can also enhance the activity of mouse LAK cells, and has a significant inhibitory effect on tumors.

Its anti-tumor (ABB) mechanism is related to its enhancement of the body's immune function and changes in cell membrane properties.

6. The effect of ZX-C anti-cancer Chinese medicine on interleukin-2 (IL-2).

The specific effective components and functions of XZ-C anti-cancer Chinese medicine or XZ-C anti-cancer Chinese medicine specific active ingredients and functions:

1. Z-C-T EBM polysaccharide

   a. At 100ug/ml, it can significantly enhance the production of human IL-2.

   b. In (EBM) 's high concentrations (2500ug/mI and 5000ug/ml), it shows inhibition. Or EBM) shows inhibitory effect at high concentration (2500ug / mI and 5000ug / ml).

   c. Epimedium, also known as Xianlingspleen, continuous subcutaneous injection for 7 days can significantly improve the ability of ConA-induced mouse thymus and spleen cells to produce IL-2.

2. Z-C-Y PEP sugar

    a. It has strong immune activity and can promote the production of IL-2.

    b. For S180 tumor mice, the IL-2 production ability of mouse spleen cells can be significantly improved.

3. Z-C--D Ginseng Polysaccharide

It has obvious promoting effect on the induction and production of IL-2 by peripheral monocytes in healthy people and patients with kidney disease, and it is in a dose-effect dependent relationship

7. The inducing and pro-inducing effect of ZX-C anti-cancer traditional Chinese medicine on interferon (IFN)

1). IFN has broad-spectrum anti-tumor effects and immunomodulatory effects.

2). IFN can inhibit tumor cell proliferation,

3). INF can activate NK cells and CTL to kill tumor cells,

4). At the same time, INF can also cooperate with TNF, IL-1, IL-2 to strengthen the anti-tumor effect

5). The effective ingredients and functions of XZ-C anti-cancer Chinese medicine:

    1)). X Z-C-Z CVQ polysaccharide

250mg/kg or 50Omg/kg can significantly increase the level of INF-y produced by mouse splenocytes.

    2)). XZ-C-D Ginseng Saponin (GS)

a. Ginseng triol saponins (PTGS) can induce human whole blood cells and monocytes to produce IFN-a and INF-y,

b. It can also restore normal IFN-y and IN-2 in tumor-bearing mice.

c. The ASH polysaccharide acute lymphocytic leukemia cell line S180 and the acute laminary leukemia cell line S7811 produced IFN titer after stimulation with

Acanthopanax senticosus polysaccharide, which was 5-10 times higher than the normal control group.

3)). XZ-C-E carboxymethyl tuckahoe polysaccharide

a. It has immune regulation, induces INF, and indirectly resists virus, reduce radiation side effects and other physiological activities.

Or, there are various physiological activities such as immune regulation, INF induction, indirect anti-virus, and reduction of radiation side effects.

b. The INF induction kinetics experiment of S180 leukemia cell line with 50mg/mi of hydrogen methyl tuckahoe polysaccharides showed that the potency of carboxymethyl tuckahoe polysaccharides in all phases was significantly higher than that of conventional induction.

4)). Z-C-G (GL)

a. It can induce IFN activity.

b. After 20h of Injecting 330mg/kg GL into mice intraperitoneally, IFN activity reached its peak.

8. **XZ-C anti-cancer Chinese medicine promotes and enhances colony stimulating factor**

a. Colony Stimulating Factor (CSF) is a type of low molecular weight glycoprotein that can stimulate the proliferation and differentiation of bone marrow hematopoietic stem cells and various mature blood cells.

b. **CSF-producing cells include mononuclear phagocytes, T cells, endothelial cells and fibroblasts.**

c. **CSF not only participates in the proliferation and differentiation of hematopoietic cells and regulates mature cells, but also plays an important role in the host's anti-tumor immunity.**

d. The effective ingredients and functions of ZX-C anti-cancer Chinese medicine:

1). XZ-C-Y PAR polysaccharide

a. It can significantly promote the production of CSF from the spleen cells of experimental mice.

b. Pokeweed Polysaccharide II 100-500ug/ml It promotes the production of CSF by splenocytes in a dose and time-dependent manner. The optimal dose is 100ug/ml, and the optimal time is 5 days.

c. Lentinan can also increase the production of CSF.

2). XZ-C-Q LBP

After injection, it can promote the secretion of CSF from mouse spleen T cells and increase the level of serum CSF activity in mice.

3). XZ-C-T EBM Epimedium

It can significantly promote ConA-induced mouse splenic lymphocyte proliferation and CSF activity.

9. XZ-C anti-cancer Chinese medicine can promote tumor necrosis factor (TNF)

a. Tumor necrosis factor (TNF) is a type of cytokine that can directly cause tumor cell death.

b. The main biological effects of TNF are:

a) Kill or inhibit tumor cells.

b) TNF can kill some tumor cells or inhibit their proliferation in vivo and in vitro.

c) XZ-C anti-tumor Chinese medicine active ingredients and functions:

1). XZ-C-Y (PEP)

1)). It can induce TNF production.

2)). PEP-1 has an inducing effect on TNF.

3)). **Inject PEP-1 80-160mg/kg into the abdominal cavity of mice, once every 4 days, then collect the peritoneal macrophages (PM), add 10ug of LPS in the culture medium to culture the PM, then take the supernatant to determine TNF and IL-1.**

It was found that PEP-1 can increase the role of LPS in assisting the production of TNF and IL-1 in parallel. The peak time of induced TNF was the 8th day after two intraperitoneal injections. Compared with the known initiator BCG, there was no difference in induced TNF.

2). XZ-C-E Carboxymethyl Tuckahoe Polysaccharide (CMP)

a. It is the main ingredient extracted from traditional Chinese medicine Poria, etc.

b. It can not only enhance the function of mouse spleen cells to produce IL-2 and phagocytes, promote the activity of T cells, B cells, NK cells, and LAK cells, but also promote the production of TNF.

c. It was proved that CMP is an effective cytokine inducer or pro-inducer.

3). XZ-C-V ABB polysaccharide

a. It can promote ConA to induce the production of TNF-b in mouse cells, and it can also induce the synthesis and secretion of TNF-a in mouse peritoneal macrophages.

b. When Niuxi polysaccharide is stimulated by 20ug/ml, the time when TNF-a reaches the peak is 2-6h after the action or, the time for TNF-a to reach the peak is 2-6h after the action,

c. Intraperitoneal injection of 100mg/kg bovine polysaccharide can promote the production of TNF-a, and the intensity of action is equivalent or comparable to that of BCG.

10. *The effect of XZ-C anti-cancer Chinese medicine on cell adhesion molecules*

Adhesion molecules are mostly glycoproteins, which are distributed on the cell surface or in the extracellular matrix. Adhesion molecules act in the form of ligand-receptor counterparts, which leads to cell-to-cell, cell-to-matrix or cell-matrix-to-cell adhesion, participate in a series of physiological and pathological processes, such as cell information transduction and activation, cell extension and movement, thrombosis, tumor metastasis, etc.

Intercellular adhesion molecule-1 (ICAM-1) is one of the adhesion molecules in the immunoglobulin superfamily.

The effect of the effective components of corn silk in XZ-C anti-cancer Chinese medicine:

Hobtematiam proves that the ethanol extract of Yushuyu has a significant inhibitory effect on endothelial cell adhesion and can effectively inhibit the expression of ICAM-1 and the endothelial cell adhesion activity mediated by TNF and LPS.

13

Research overview of XZ-C immunomodulatory anti-cancer Chinese medication

The Experimental Study

In 1985, it was to conduct the systematic follow-up statistics on more than 3,000 patients who had undergone chest and abdomen cancer surgery performed by the author, and it was found that most of the patients had recurred or metastasized within 2-3 years.

In order to reduce the recurrence rate and increase the treatment rate, it is necessary to conduct basic clinical research. Without breakthroughs in basic research, it is difficult to improve clinical efficacy.

The existing anti-cancer drugs are cytotoxic drugs that kill both tumor cells and normal cells, with great side effects. The existing anticancer drugs such as vinblastine, which are discovered from traditional Chinese medicine, are alkaloids proposed from vinca. It has been used clinically as an anticancer drug, but it also kills normal cells and has serious side effects.

However, we want anticancer agents that have fewer side effects, are effective when taken orally, and can enhance patients' physical strength and resistance so that it was to carry out a scientific research design.

a. It was planned to find new anti-cancer drugs from natural drugs through animal experiments in cancer-bearing mice;

b. It was to look for anti-metastasis and anti-relapse drugs,

c. And look for only cancer cells but not normal cells Chinese medicine, looking for new drugs that can adjust the regulatory relationship between the host and the tumor.

According to the theory of cell proliferation cycle, the anticancer agent must be able to be applied continuously for a long time, so that the cancer foci can be continuously immersed in the anticancer agent for a long time, so as to prevent its cell division and prevent recurrence and metastasis.

It must be carried out over a long period of time and for a long period of time to control the existing cancer foci and prevent the formation of new cancer cells.

However, the currently used anticancer drugs cannot be used continuously for a long time due to the large side effects. They can only be applied in a short period of time.

The existing anticancer drugs have the side effects of suppressing immune function, suppressing bone marrow hematopoietic function, suppressing thymus, and suppressing bone marrow.

__The formation and development of cancer is due to the patient's reduced immunity and loss of immune monitoring.__

__Therefore, all anti-cancer drugs must increase immunity and protect immune organs, rather than suppress immune drugs.__

To this end, our laboratory has carried out the following experimental research on selecting new anti-cancer and anti-metastasis drugs from Chinese medicine:

(1) *__Using the method of in vitro culturing of cancer cells to carry out the screening experimental research on the antitumor rate of Chinese herbal medicine__*

In vitro screening test:

The tumor cells were cultured in vitro to observe the direct damage of drugs to tumor cells.

1. method

(1) Preparation of crude drug preparations:

Dry crude drug, add 60 times of water, heat to extract and filter, and distill the filtrate to dryness under reduced pressure to form a crude powder, ready to use.

It was to dry crude drug, then to add 60 times water, later it was to heat the drug to extract and filter; the filtrate fluid can be stressed reliever and became distillation until it become dry to form a coarse powder, and it can be applied.

(2) In-test tube screening test:

Ehrlich ascites carcinoma (EAC), or sarcoma 180 (S180), or ascites hepatoma (H22), or cervical cancer cell 1X105/ml, fetal bovine serum 10%, crude drug 500ug/ml, this ratio Inject 20 ml of the solution and place it in a 10 X 15 cm culture dish at 37°C for 134 hours. Then compare the number of surviving cells with the control group to determine the inhibition rate of cell proliferation caused by cytotoxicity.

It was to prepare for 1X105/ml of Ehrlich ascites carcinoma (EAC), or sarcoma 180 (S180), or ascites hepatoma (H22), or cervical cancer cell, and 10% of fetal bovine serum, 500ug/ml of crude drug, and then based on this ratio, it was to inject 20 ml of the solution at this ratio into a 10 X 15 cm petri dish and place it at 37°C for 134 hours.

Then compare the number of surviving cells with the control group to determine the inhibition rate of cell proliferation caused by cytotoxicity.

(3) Drug screening:

It was to put crude drugs into the test tubes for culturing human cancer cells to observe whether they have an inhibitory effect on cancer cells.

We will carry out in vitro screening tests one by one of 200 Chinese herbal medicines that traditional Chinese medicine considers to have anti-cancer effects.

Also under the same conditions, normal human fiber cells were cultured to determine the cytotoxicity of the drug to such cells and then compare.

2. Experimental results

Among the 200 crude drugs screened in our laboratory through animal experiments, 48 were screened to have certain or even excellent inhibitory effects on the proliferation of cancer cells, with a tumor inhibition rate of over 90%. However, there are also some commonly used Chinese medicines that are generally considered to be anti-cancer. After experiments, they have no anti-cancer effect or have little effect.

In addition, 50 kinds of traditional Chinese medicines have an inhibition rate below 30%, such as Weilingxian, Prunella vulgaris, Dilong, August Zha, Digupi, Wild Rose, etc.

(2) *It was to manufacture animal models and conduct experimental research on the anti-tumor rate of Chinese herbal medicine in cancer-bearing animals*

1. In vivo tumor suppression screening test
The tumor-bearing animal model:

240 Kunming mice were used in each batch of experiments, divided into 8 groups, 30 in each group; or each batch of experiments uses 240 Kunming mice, divided into 8 groups, each with 30 mice; the first, the second, the third, the fourth, the fifth, and the sixth experimental group for one chinese medicine in each group, and the seventh group as the blank control group, the 8th group uses 5-FU or CTX as the control group. The whole group of mice was subcutaneously inoculated with EAC or S180 or H22 cancer cells 1X107/ml in the right anterior armpit. Mung bean-sized tumor nodules were grown under the skin 3 days later.

After 24 hours of inoculation, each rat was orally fed with crude drug powder.

According to body weight 1000mg/kg, once a day, it was to feed for 8 weeks, daily measurement of body weight and tumor nodule size, after 8 weeks, 20 animals in each group were sacrificed for measuring body weight and tumor weight, and it was to weigh the organs such as liver, spleen, lung, and thymus, etc and slice them; it was to observe the organization or tissue situation and understand the transfer situation.

The other 10 tumor-bearing experimental mice were fed the selected Chinese medicine for a long time. It was to observe survival period, toxicity and side effects, calculate prolonged survival rate, calculate tumor inhibition rate; the experiment period of each batch (that is, the screening of each Chinese medicine) is 3 months. In each batch of experiments, 6 Chinese medicines or 6 prescriptions can be screened and studied simultaneously. This set of experiments can simultaneously obtain the screening results of 6 medicines.

The institute can conduct 3 experimental group experiments at the same time, and each batch of 3 master's or doctoral students can manage 1 experimental group to simultaneously study 18 single-flavor Chinese medicines or 18 prescription tumor suppression experiments.

One year It can carry out and complete the 72-flavored single-flavored Chinese medicine screening experiment in vivo in tumor-bearing mice.

In this way, we conducted 4 consecutive years of experimental research, and also conducted 3 years of experimental research on the pathogenesis and metastasis and recurrence mechanisms of tumor-bearing mice, as well as experimental research to explore why the cancer caused the death of the host.

1,000 tumor-bearing animal models are used every year, and nearly 6,000 tumor-bearing animal models have been made in 4 years.

After the death of each experimental mouse, the pathological anatomy of liver, spleen, lung, chest, spleen, and kidney were performed, and a total of 20,000 of slides or sections were performed. The multiple sections were taken to explore and find the tiny pathogens causing cancer.

Microcirculation microscopy was used to observe the establishment of tumor microvessels and microcirculation in 100 tumor-bearing mice.

Through experimental research, we discovered for the first time in China that the traditional Chinese medicine TG has a significant effect on inhibiting tumor microvessel formation. It has been used in clinical anti-metastasis treatment for 200 cases of patients, and the efficacy is under observation.

2. Discuss

(1). **Through experimental research, it was to put forward new thinking, new understanding, new concept and new strategy for anti-cancer:**

After 7 years, it was to make more than 6000 tumor-bearing animal models, and to perform the In vivo tumor suppression test of anti-cancer, anti-metastasis and anti-relapse for 200 kinds of natural Chinese herbal medication, and it was to produce the ideas, understandings and experiences that traditional anti-cancer work need to update concepts, thinking, and traditional principles and methods.

Through the use of tumor-bearing animal models to conduct scientific, objective and rigorous experimental screening, analysis, and evaluation of 200 Chinese medicines with anti-cancer curative effects in traditional Chinese medicine literature, only 48 have good anti-cancer effects.

The 200 kinds of Chinese herbal medicines selected in the experiment were selected from more than 10 famous anticancer prescriptions of Chinese medicine. They are also commonly used drugs with anticancer effects reported in Chinese medicine journals and literature.

Why the experimental research results show that there are 152 kinds of traditional Chinese medicines that have no tumor inhibition rate or low anti-cancer effect. It may be that the traditional Chinese medicine literature does not distinguish the tumors and symptoms of traditional Chinese medicine from cancer in modern medicine.

The 48 kinds of traditional Chinese medicines selected by animal experiments in this group have a good tumor inhibition rate. After optimized combination and repeated experiments, the ZX-Cl-10 immunomodulatory anti-cancer Chinese medicine preparation was formed. It has been clinically verified for 30 years, and more than 12,000 cancer patients have been applied for verification, and good results have been achieved.

Through this group of experiments to screen the research results, we realize that traditional Chinese medicine prescriptions are obtained from many years of experience. It is a complex of various crude drugs composed of disease symptoms. From the perspective of TCM literature, the symptoms of disease and accumulation seem similar to cancer.

Using traditional Chinese medicine to treat the disease, sometimes the symptoms can be improved, but not all cancers. Generally speaking, it has no effect on cancer, so we should use modern scientific methods to verify, observe, and re-evaluate the anti-cancer or carcinogenicity of various crude drugs in Chinese medicine prescriptions to avoid the unscientific parts of traditional Chinese medicine.

In the drug screening experiment, we also found that the single crude drug is not as effective as the optimal combination of several crude drugs.

It may be that the single crude drug only has an effect on the inhibition of tumor proliferation, and the compound prescription of the optimized combination of multi-morbidity crude drug not only inhibits the tumor proliferation of tumor-bearing mice, but also enhances physical strength, improves immunity, and promotes the production of cancer suppressor factors and protect normal cells.

Since 1992, after 7 years of scientific research, XZ-C1-10 immunomodulatory anti-cancer Chinese medicine has been screened and formed.

This medicine has the effects of anti-cancer, strengthening the body and eliminating evil, clearing heat and detoxification, and promoting blood circulation and removing stasis and disease.

From experimental research to clinical verification, and from clinical to experiment. We organized and established a joint anti-cancer and anti-cancer cooperation team. The cooperative group has an experimental research base and a clinical application verification base, the former is in the medical school and the laboratory of the Medical University, and the latter is in the clinical medical department of the National Cooperation Group of Anti-tumor Research and Combination of Chinese and Western Medicine.

From experiment to clinic, it is applied to clinic on the basis of successful experimental research. In the process of clinical application, new problems were discovered, basic experimental research was conducted, and the new experimental results were applied to clinical verification. It is such experiment→clinical→re-experiment→re-clinical, and it is continuously cyclically increasing.

After 30 years of clinical practice, the understanding has also been continuously rising.

Summarization, analysis, reflection, and evaluation have risen to theory, and it is to put forward new understandings, new concepts, new thinking, new strategies, new treatment routes and plans.

The research experience of the collaborative group is:

① It is to build the road of joint research by professors, experts, postgraduates and scientific research collaboration of universities and colleges, to promote scientific research collaboration, and to attach importance to organizing the scientific research and technical strength of all parties and to enrich anti-cancer power.

② Anti-cancer and anti-cancer should make use of national advantages and give full play to the advantages of traditional Chinese herbal medicine, which is in line with my country's national conditions.

③ Basic research is important, but application and development research are more important.

It should be from basic research→ application research→ development research, the focus is on application and efficacy.

It should pay attention to improving the quality of life of cancer patients, improving symptoms, and prolonging survival.

④ It was to restore outpatient medical records (After the Cultural Revolution, Hubei Province cancelled the preservation of medical records in outpatient clinics and delegated medical records to patients).

It was to complete and detailed outpatient medical records in order to obtain complete clinical verification data for analysis, statistics and follow-up.

Usually 80%-90% of patients are treated in outpatient clinics, and 10%-20% of patients are treated in hospitals. The current inpatient medical records are preserved and clinical data can be analyzed and researched, while 80%-90% of patients are treated in outpatient clinics.

Without the outpatient medical records, analysis, statistics, and follow-up of outpatients' curative effect in outpatient clinics cannot be performed.

Inpatient medical records can only observe short-term effects, while keeping outpatient medical records can observe long-term effects.

The restoration of outpatient medical records is conducive to outpatient clinical research to improve the quality of medical care.

(2). *The experimental work to find new anti-cancer, anti-metastasis, and anti-relapse drugs from natural medicines:*

Its purpose is to screen out long-term oral anticancer drugs without drug resistance, no toxic side effects, and high selectivity.

As we all know, although the current anticancer drugs can inhibit cell proliferation, due to their severe side effects, many patients have to stop the drug during use, and cancer cells re-proliferate after stopping the drug, and began to have resistance.

A well-known anti-cancer drug such as azmetaquinone, which was viewed from the cancer cell tissue culture, the drug resistance can be 20,000 times, usually only a few milligrams was used before drug resistance, but when drug resistance occurs, this dose will not work, so the dose must be increased. However, when this anticancer drug is increased to 10 times the amount, the patient will be fatal.

Therefore, the resistance of cancer cells to anticancer drugs and the side effects of anticancer drugs on the host are long-term troublesome problems.

a. The purpose of the new drugs we are looking for is to avoid these shortcomings.

b. **The purpose is to screen out anticancer drugs that are neither tolerable nor toxic and side-effects, and highly selective. It is best to take long-term oral anticancer drugs**.

c. Western medicine anti-cancer drugs have a single component, although they are effective in small amounts, they inhibit 100% of normal cells, and their side effects are quite large.

Some existing anti-cancer drugs are extracted from traditional Chinese medicines, such as vincristine, camptothecin, and Colchicine, these alkaloids are similar to traditional anticancer drugs, that is, they are effective in small amounts, but are very toxic.

Whether can you find an anti-cancer Chinese medicine from Chinese medicine that can inhibit the growth of cancer cells without killing normal cells or not?

After several years of experimental screening, we finally found that many Chinese medicines have ideal anti-cancer effects. Often when the dose is 500ug/ml, it has an inhibitory effect on cancer cells.

ZX-C1 and XZ-C4 drugs that can inhibit cancer cells 100% without harming normal cells have also been found.

**Among them, XZ-C1, XZ-C4 and XZ-C8 also proliferate normal cells and improve the immune function of the host. This is a major feature of Chinese medicine in anti-cancer.**

For example, the anti-cancer effect of XZ-C Chinese medicine varies with the concentration of the dose:

a. At 250ug/ml, it can only inhibit 60% of cancer cells;

b. When 125ug/ml, the inhibition rate is zero;

c. Type A drugs are effective in small amounts, such as vinblastine, small polyalkaloids in coptis, alkaloids in myrobalan, but they also have an inhibitory effect on normal cell proliferation, which is the same as traditional anticancer drugs;

d. Type B drugs are other anti-cancer Chinese medicines, which are effective at high concentrations, that is, they have no effect on inhibiting cancer cells in small amounts. The dose-effect is proportional, and the larger the dose, the better the effects are, such as XZ-C1-A-B.

3. Clinical effect verification

Over the past 10 years, we have used experimental crude drugs in the clinic, and we can see that the clinical effects of XZ-C drugs are quite different, that is, after the administration of type B drugs for a considerable period of time, the cancer cells neither proliferate nor shrink, while the patient's Energetic became stronger. After a few months, the physical strength became stronger, and the cancer began to shrink slowly. This is probably not a toxic effect on cancer cells.

Instead, it creates an environment that is not conducive to the proliferation of cancer cells in the body.

When it was to have the long-term administration, there is no toxic accumulation effect on normal cells. Many patients have taken XZ-C1+ZX-C4 for 3-5 years without recurrence and metastasis, and no side effects. Long-term massive administration has received unexpectedly good results.

The different types of XZ-C preparations are given according to different types of cancer, such as digestive tract cancer, lung cancer, uterine cancer, etc., must be formulated according to symptoms so that it will receive good results.

It is different from traditional decoctions, what we give is a mixture of various single crude drugs passed through a 100-mesh sieve to form a compound, not a decoction compound, but a mixture, which can maintain the pharmacology of each crude drug Characteristics, **there are no side effects when taken for a long time, it is very meaningful to explore the use of crude drugs.**

In actual clinical practice, will there be any problems with long-term use?

The patient has two conditions:

There is no abnormality in taking a considerable amount, and the effect appears slowly.

Many patients have been taking XZ-C4 for 3-5 years, and their mental condition and appetite are good, their physical strength is restored, their physical fitness is enhanced, their condition is stable, and their condition is good.

A crude product with a clinical daily amount of about 20g, of which the main drug is an anticancer drug, accounting for about 10% (equivalent to 40g crude drug). This is quite different from the amount of traditional Chinese medicine, which is a large dose.

After taking the medicine, when will the effect appear?

Generally 1-3 months are the highest peak. Therefore, if the patient can survive for more than 6 months, about 90% of the symptoms can be significantly changed, 50% of the patients stop cancer proliferation, and about 80% can see the effect of prolonging the survival period.

It is of great significance that XZ-C1-4 crude drug products have a good analgesic effect.

Liver cancer and pancreatic cancer have severe pain in the middle and late stages.

Patients who have used this crude drug for more than one month say that there is almost no pain, and they can even avoid the injection of painkillers, which is really incredible.

The extract of single crude drug and the extract of mixed crude drug have almost no change in effect. But when the traditional compound decoction is used, the effect is slightly worse, which may be due to the interaction of the drugs.

As far as cancer treatment is concerned, it is better to use a mixture.

Please note that there are also crude drugs that can promote the reproduction of cancer cells and inhibit normal cells, especially mineral and animal crude drugs, such as viper and velvet antler. Even small amounts can promote the above-mentioned adverse effects. Centipedes can damage the renal tubules.

Anticancer properties of natural medicines:

Sato Zhaohiko believes that there are three categories:

One is that the contained ingredients have cancer-killing effects, such as vinblastine.

The second is that some medicines such as purple ganoderma and evodia polysaccharides. **Because of its immune-enhancing effect, it is very popular as an immunotherapy**, but it has a limit. It is almost helpless in the development and terminal stages of cancer, but it can be used as a good auxiliary drug because of its few side effects.

The third is the above-mentioned type B anticancer drugs. Its mechanism of action is not yet clear. At high concentrations, it can inhibit the proliferation of cancer cells, but does not inhibit normal cells and has fewer toxic side effects.

It can be taken for a long time, but it does not kill cancer or promote immune function. It can be considered as a new type of medicine.

In the past 10 years, due to coronary heart disease, the author rarely went out and did not attend academic conferences in other provinces or places. I have time to sit down for a long time and do concrete animal experiments and clinical verification research work, and I have gained a lot.

With in-depth research, a large number of patients are contacted every month, and many materials that are not recorded in books and documents are obtained. I have a deep understanding of the epidemiology, clinical symptoms, evolution and progress of signs, and in many cases after analysis, evaluation, and reflection.

Sit down and conduct a series of animal experiments on cancer prevention and anti-cancer basic research with graduate students and laboratory researchers.

14

The experimental and clinical observation of XZ-C immune regulation and control anti-cancer Chinese medicine for the treatment of malignant tumors

In order to find anti-cancer Chinese medicine that has anti-cancer curative effect *without toxic and side effects to the body*, our Institute of Surgical Oncology has screened 200 kinds of Chinese herbal medicines with anti-cancer effects recorded in Chinese medicine books one by one for the anti-tumor effects of solid tumors in tumor-bearing animal models in 4 years.

After a long-term batch of in vivo tumor suppression animal experiments, 48 kinds of Chinese herbal medicines *that have a good tumor suppression rate (cancer inhibiting rate) and prolong survival, protect immune organs and significantly improve immune function* have been screened.

According to dialectics of the disease clinical condition and the treatment principles of strengthening the body and removing the evil, softening hard parts and dispelling the masses, and anti-cancer promotion and immunity, the selected anti-cancer drugs are combined into two compounds XZ-C1 and XZ-C4 that have better anti-cancer effects than each single agent.

The initial screening was a cancer-suppressing animal experiment for each single herbal medicine. Now we are going further to conduct further experimental research on the anti-tumor effect of these two groups of compound on solid tumors in tumor-bearing mice.

1. Animal Experimental Research

1). Materials and methods

(1) Experimental animals, 260 pure Kunming mice, half male and half, weighing 21±2g, 8-10 weeks old.

(2) Tumor strain and inoculation:

Liver cancer H22 tumor line, take fresh tumor body of tumor-bearing mice to make a single cell suspension, after staining and counting the cancer cells $((1\times10^6/ml)$, 0.2ml of normal saline for cancer cells is placed on the right anterior axillary of each mouse Subcutaneous vaccination.

(3) Drug and experimental grouping:

The traditional Chinese medicine XZ-C$_1$ and XZ-C$_4$ are both developed and developed by the Anti-Cancer Collaborative Group. The former is a mixture, the latter is a powder (infusion), and the chemotherapy control drug used in the chemotherapy group is cyclophosphamide (CTX).

The experiment grouping:

The H22 cancer cell transplanted animals were randomly divided into four groups:

1). In the traditional Chinese medicine XZ-C$_1$ group (90 mice), mice were intragastrically administered once a day for 24 hours after cancer cell transplantation or inoculation, 0.8ml each time per mouse, which is equivalent to 1.4mg crude drug.

2). Traditional Chinese medicine XZ-C$_4$ group ((90 animals), the dosage and gastric administration method are the same as above.

3). Chemotherapy group (50 animals), starting from the next day after cancer cell transplantation, intragastric administration of CTX 50mg/kg body weight was performed every other day.

4). For the control group (30 mice), starting from the next day after cancer cell transplantation, 0.8ml of normal saline was administered daily.

(4) Observation index:

    a. The weight of the mouse was measured every 3 days,

    b. The diameter of the tumor was measured with a vernier caliper,

    c. the immune function was measured, and the blood picture was determined.

Half of each group is group A:

    a. in the tumor-bearing experiment, the mice are executed periodically in batches,

    b. the tumor pieces are separated and the tumor weight is calculated, and the tumor inhibition rate is calculated.

    c. The tumor was made pathological section,

    d. and a few specimens were observed for ultrastructure.

The other half of each group is group B:

    a. tumor-bearing experimental mice, long-term infusion or administration of medicine, until they died naturally. After the mice died, the tumor mass was separated and weighed, and the long-term tumor inhibition rate and life extension rate were calculated.

2). The experimental results

(1) The anti-tumor effect of XZ-C Chinese medicine on H22 mice bearing liver cancer:

The tumor inhibition rate <u>of XZ-C1 was</u> 40% in the second week, 45% in the fourth week, and 58% in the sixth week.

The tumor inhibition rate <u>of XZ-C4 was</u> 53% in the second week, 68% in the fourth week, and 70% in the sixth week. (P<0.01)

In the second week of CTX medication, the tumor inhibition rate was 45%. The tumor inhibition rate was 45% in the 4th week and 49% in the 6th week (Figure 1, Figure 2).

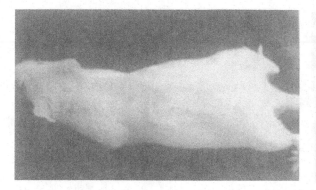 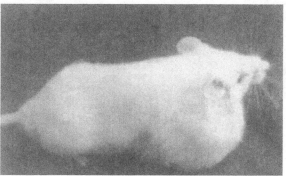

Figure 1	Figure 2
XZ-C1, XZ-C4 treatment group 30 days after inoculation of liver cancer H22	Control group 30 days after inoculation of liver cancer H22

(2) The effect of XZ-C Chinese medicine on the survival time of H22 mice bearing liver cancer

The average survival days of XZ-C1, XZ-C4, and CTX groups were higher than those of the saline control group (P<0.01), and XZ-C Chinese medicine had a significant effect on prolonging survival.

Compared with the control group, the life extension rate of XZ-C1 group was 35%, the life extension rate of XZ-C4 group was 200%, and the life extension rate of CTX group was 9.8%.

Both XZ-C1 and CTX groups in group B died within 75 days.

In the XZ-C4 group, 6 bearing mice were still alive after 7 months.

(3) XZ-C1 and XZ-C4 Chinese medicines both increase immune function.

a. XZ-C4 can significantly improve immune function, increase white blood cells and red blood cells, *has no effect on liver and kidney function, and has no damage to liver and kidney slices*. CTX reduces white blood cells and reduces immune function. Kidney slices have kidney damage.

The thymus in the control group was significantly atrophy (Figure 3). The thymus in the XZ-C1 and XZ-C4 treatment groups did not shrink and was slightly hypertrophy (Figure 4).

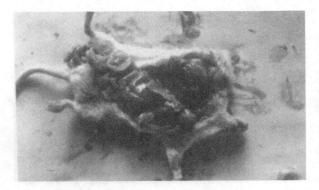
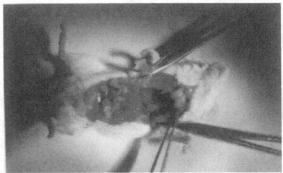

Figure 3 XZ-C4 treatment group	Figure 4 Control group
Thirty days after hepatocarcinoma H22 inoculation, the thymus gland is obviously hypertrophy	Thirty days after hepatocellular carcinoma H22 inoculation, the thymus glands are obviously swollen.

b. Pathological section of control thymus:

Thymic cortex is atrophy, cells are sparse, and blood vessels are congested (Figure 5).

In the XZ-C4 treatment group Thymus pathological section showed thickened thymic cortex, dense lymphocytes, increased epithelial reticulocytes, and increased thymic corpuscles (Figure 6).

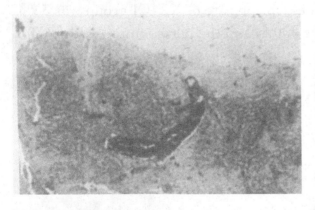
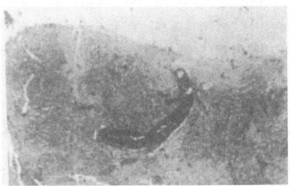

Figure 5 Pathological section of thymus in tumor-bearing control group HEx100 cortical atrophy The lymphocytes are significantly reduced, Cortical area forms a lymphocyte empty zone, blood stasis in blood vessel	Figure 6 Thymus in XZ-4 treatment group HEX100 Thymus cortex medulla is thickened and lymphocytes are highly dense

2. Clinical application observation

1). Clinical data

(1) XZ-C immunomodulatory anti-cancer Chinese medicine combined with Chinese and Western medicine was used to treat 4698 cases of stage III, IV or metastatic or recurrent cancer, including 3051 males and 1647 females in integrated Chinese and Western Medicine Anti-cancer Research National Collaborative Group Hubei Group, Anti-tumor Metastasis and Recurrence Research Laboratory and Shuguang Oncology Specialist Outpatient Department, from 1994 to November 2002. The youngest is 11 years old, the oldest is 86 years old, and the age at high incidence is 40-69 years old.

All patients in the whole group were diagnosed by histopathology or B-ultrasound, CT, MRI imaging. According to the International Anti-Cancer Alliance's staging standards, all cases are stage III or above in advanced stage patients.

There are 1021 cases of liver cancer in this group, including 694 cases of primary liver cancer and 327 cases of metastatic liver cancer; 752 cases of lung cancer, including 699 cases of primary lung cancer, 53 cases of metastatic lung cancer; 668 cases of gastric cancer, 624 cases of esophagus and cardia cancer, 328 cases of rectal and anal cancer, 442 cases of colon cancer, 368 cases of breast cancer, 74 cases of pancreatic cancer, 30 cases of bile duct cancer, 43 cases of retroperitoneal tumors, 38 cases of ovarian cancer, 9 cases of cervical cancer, 11 cases of brain tumor, 34 cases of thyroid cancer, 38 cases of nasopharyngeal cancer, 9 cases of melanoma, 27 cases of kidney cancer, 48 cases of bladder cancer, 13 cases of leukemia, and 47 cases of supraclavicular lymph node metastasis Cases, 35 cases of various sarcomas, 39 cases of other malignant tumors.

(2) Drugs and methods of administration:

The treatment principle is to strengthen the body and eliminate the evil, soften the firmness and dispel lumps, and tonic the qi and blood.

XZ-C1 is a mixture, 150ml daily, XZ-C4 is a powder (granule), 10g daily.

According to the dialectical rules of the disease conditions or syndrome differentiation, solid tumors or metastatic masses should be treated with anticancer powder orally and anticancer swelling cream externally. For those with pain, apply topical anticancer pain relief cream.

For jaundice and ascites, add Tuihuang Decoction or Xiaoshui Decoction.

(3) Efficacy evaluation:

It is not only pay attention to short-term efficacy and imaging indicators, but also pay more attention to long-term efficacy, survival, quality of life, and immune indicators.

It was to pay attention to the changes in the subjective symptoms during the medication. If the subjective symptoms improve and last for more than 1 month, it is effective, otherwise it is invalid. The improvement of the quality of life (Kafler score) needs to be effective for more than 1 month, otherwise it is invalid.

The curative effect evaluation criteria of solid tumor masses are divided into 4 levels according to the change of tumor size:

Grade I: the mass disappeared;

Grade II: The mass is reduced by 1/2;

Grade III: The lump becomes soft;

Grade IV: No change or enlargement of the mass.

5). Treatment result

(1) Improved symptoms, improved quality of life, and prolonged survival:

Among 4277 patients with intermediate and advanced cancer who took XZ-C immunoregulatory Chinese medicine for more than 3 months, the medical records have detailed curative effect observation records, see Table 15-1. Comprehensively improve the patient's quality of life, see Table 1.

Table 1 General data of 4277 cases of recurrence and metastasis

	Liver cancer	Lung cancer	Stomach cancer	Esophagus and Cardia Cancer	Rectal and anal cancer	Colon cancer	Breast cancer	Pancreatic cancer
Number of cases (cases)	1021	752	668	624	328	442	368	74
men :women Lesion	4:1	4.4:1	2.25:1	3.1:1	1:1	2.1:1	All of female	3.2:1
Primary	694 (68.8%)	699(93.9%)						
Metastasis	327 (31.2%)	53 (6.1%)						

Common metastatic sites in this group	Lung metastasis (2%) From stomach (27.2%) From esophagus and cardia(19.5%) From the rectum (31.2%)	Supraclavicular lymph node metastasis (11.6%) Brain metastasis(3.1%) Bone metastasis (4.6%)	Metastasis to liver (23.8%) Lung metastasis (3%) peritoneal metastasis (29.1%) Supraclavicular (6.1%)	Supraclavicular metastasis (13.1%) Metastasis liver(8.3%)	Recurrence rate (14.6%) Metastasis liver (7.0%)	Metastasis to liver (16.0%) Peritoneal metastasis (6.0%)	Supraclavicular lymph node metastasis (17.5%) Extra-Axillary lymph node metastasis (15.0%) Bone metastasis (5.0%)	Metastasis to liver (11.7%) Post-Peritoneal metastasis (39.1%)
Age Peak age(yr) (%)	30-39 (76.2)	50-69 (71.6)	40-49 (73.4)	40-69(75.2)	30-69(88.0)	30-69(88.0)	40-59(65.9)	40-59(70.0)
Minaxium age(yr)	11	20	17	27	27	27	29	34
Maximium age(yr)	86	80	77	78	76	76	80	68

154

Table 2 Observation of curative effect of 4277 cases to comprehensively improve the quality of life of advanced cancer patients

Improvement	Mental Or spirit will	appetite	Strengthen Improvement	Generally things get better	Weight	Long sleep gets better	Improving activities' ability to motivate and motion limit relief	Take care of your own life and walk as usual	Resumption of work from : light physical work
Number of cases	4071	3986	2450.	479	2938	1005	1038	3220	479
(%)	95.2	93.2	57.3	11.2	68.7	23.5	24.3	75.3	11.2

All patients in this group were in the middle and late stages, and all had different degrees of symptom improvement after taking the medicine, with an effective rate of 93.2%.

In terms of improving the quality of life (according to the Karnofsky scoring standard), the average score is 50 before medication, and the average score is 80 after medication.

All patients in this group have metastasis and dysfunction of different tissues and organs above stage III.

Previous statistics for such patients have reported that the median survival time is about 6 months. The longest cases in this group have reached 11 years, and the average survival time of the remaining cases is more than 1 year.

One case of primary liver cancer in the left lobe of the liver, recurred in the right liver after resection, and had been treated with XZ-C alone for 11 years;

Another case of liver cancer has been taking XZ-C for 10 and a half years;

In 2 cases of liver cancer, there were multiple cancers in the liver. After taking XZ-C for half a year, the cancers completely disappeared after 2 CT reexaminations, and they have been stable for half a year.

One case of double kidney cancer had extensive metastasis to the abdominal cavity after one side was resected. After taking XZ-C medicine, he has completely returned to work.

Three cases of lung cancer could not be cut through open chest examination, and they had been taking XZ-C medicine for 3 and a half years.

2 cases of remnant gastric cancer have taken XZ-C medicine for 8 years;

3 cases of rectal cancer recurrence took XZ-C medicine for 3 years.

One case of breast cancer metastasis to the liver and ribs has been taking medicine for 8 years.

One case of recurrence of bladder cancer after renal cancer surgery, disappeared after taking XZ-C drug for 9 and a half years.

The above cases are all patients in the middle and late stages who cannot undergo surgery, radiotherapy or chemotherapy. They are treated with XZ-C drugs only and no other drugs are used.

So far, I still come to the clinic every month for review and medicine. After long-term medication, the condition is controlled in a stable state, so that the body and the tumor can maintain a balance state for a long time, and a better survival with the tumor can be obtained. The symptoms of the patient are improved, the quality of life is improved, and the survival period is prolonged.

(2) For 84 cases of solid masses and 56 cases of patients with metastatic supraclavicular lymphadenopathy, the XZ-C series and external application of XZ-C3 anti-cancer softening knot ointment have achieved good results, see Table 3.

Table 3 Changes of 84 cases of solid masses and 56 cases of metastatic nodules after external application of XZ-C ointment

	Solid mass				Swollen supraclavicular lymph nodes in the neck			
	Disappear	shrink by ½	Soften	without change	Disappear	shrink by ½	Soften	without change
The number of case	18	28	32	12	12	22	14	8
(%)	14.2	33.3	38.0	14.2	21.4	39.2	25.0	14. 2
Total effective rate			85.7				85.7	

(3) 298 cases of cancer pain patients took XZ-C internally and externally applied XZ-C anticancer analgesic ointment to achieve significant analgesic effects, see Table 4.

Table 4 Pain relief after oral administration of XZ-C medicine and external application of XZ-C anticancer pain relief ointment in 298 patients

Clinical manifestations	Pain			
	Mild relief	Significantly reduced	Disappear	Invalid
Number of cases	52	139	93	14
(%)				
Total effective rate (%)	17.3	46.8	31.2	4.7
		95.3		

3. The experiment and clinical efficacy of XZ-C immune regulation and control anti-cancer Chinese medicine

1). The effect of XZ-C1-4 anti-cancer Chinese medicine on tumor-inhibition of H22 tumor-bearing mice

It was found that the tumor inhibition rate of H22 tumor-bearing mice was observed after 2 weeks, 4 weeks, and 6 weeks, and the tumor inhibition rate increased with the extension of the medication time. The tumor inhibition rate of XZ-C4 was as high as 70% at the 6th week.

After the subsequent 2 repeated tests, the results are stable, indicating that the anti-tumor effect of Chinese medicine is slow and gradually increasing, that is, the anti-tumor effect is positively correlated with the cumulative dose of Chinese medicine.

The effect of XZ-C1, XZ-C4 anti-cancer Chinese medicine on the survival period of H22 tumor-bearing mice:

The experimental results prove that XZ-C1, XZ-C4 anti-cancer Chinese medicine can significantly prolong the survival time of tumor-bearing mice, especially XZ-C4, **significantly prolonging its survival time by more than 200%, not only that, XZ-C4 can also significantly improve the body Immune function, protection of immune organs, protection of bone marrow, alleviation of side effects of chemotherapy and radiotherapy drugs, no side effects have been seen by mice for up to 12 months**.

The above experimental research provides a beneficial basis for clinical application.

2). The clinical efficacy

    a. On the basis of experimental research, it has been applied to various types of clinical cancers since 1994, mostly in patients with stage III and IV or above, namely:

    b. Advanced cancer that cannot be removed by exploratory surgery;

    c. Those with advanced cancer who have lost the indication for surgery;

    d. Those who have recently or long-term metastasis or recurrence after various cancer operations;

e. Liver metastasis, lung metastasis, brain metastasis of various advanced cancers, or combined with cancerous pleural effusion and cancerous ascites;

f. All kinds of cancer limit resection surgery, that is, the exploration can only do gastrointestinal anastomosis or colostomy, but cancer cannot be removed;

g. Patients who are not suitable for surgery, radiotherapy, chemotherapy, etc.

XZ-C1 and XZ-C4 anti-cancer Chinese medicines have been clinically used for more than 30 years and through systematically observed it was to have achieved obvious curative effects, and no toxic side effects have been seen after long-term use.

Clinical observations have proved that XZ-C1, XZ-C4 anti-cancer Chinese medicine can comprehensively improve the quality of life of patients with advanced cancer, improve overall immunity, control cancer cell proliferation, and consolidate and enhance long-term efficacy.

Oral and external application of XZ-C medicine has a good effect on softening and reducing body surface metastatic tumors. When combined with intermediary or intubation drug pump treatment, it can protect the liver, kidney, bone marrow hematopoietic system and immune organs, and improve immunity.

3). Z-C Anticancer Pain Relief Ointment has good analgesic effect

Pain is a more obvious and painful symptom for patients with advanced cancer.

General analgesics have little effect on cancer pain, and narcotic analgesics are addictive and dependent.

XZ-C Anticancer Pain Relief Ointment has a strong analgesic effect and a long maintenance time. After 298 cases of clinical verification, the effective rate is 78.0%, and the total effective rate is 95.3%.

Repeated use has no obvious side effects, no addiction, and stable analgesic effect. It is an effective treatment method for cancer patients to relieve pain and improve the quality of life.

Through experimental research and clinical verification, our experience is:

Traditional Chinese medicine with Chinese characteristics has unique advantages in tumor treatment, such as a strong overall concept, the outstanding role of conditioning, mild side effects, it can relieve pain, relieve symptoms, significantly improve the patient's

quality of life, adjust the body's immune function and overall disease resistance, and improve the therapeutic effect.

4. The research of the cytokine induced by XZ-C4 anti-cancer traditional Chinese medicine

XZ-C anti-cancer Chinese medicine can induce endogenous cytokines

(1) According to experimental research, XZ-C4 has a variety of immune enhancement effects, and is closely related to the induction of endogenous cytokines.

(2) XZ-C4 can inhibit the reduction of white blood cells, granulocytes and platelets.

(3) XZ-C4 not only has a direct effect on the production of granulocyte macrophage colony stimulating factor (GM-CSF) through interleukin-1ß (IL-1 ß), but also can enhance tumor necrosis factor (TNF), interferon (IFN)) And other cytokines, the latter may be an indirect mechanism of action.

(4) In cancer patients, Th1 cytokine that regulates cellular immune function has decreased, while XZ-C4 can increase it. It is effective for anemia and leukopenia after chemotherapy.

(5) The experimental analysis found that XZ-C4 not only protects the bone marrow, but also has a direct effect on the differentiation of cancer cells through cytokines.

In short, XZ-C4 exhibits various cytokines due to autocrine, thereby inducing cancer cell differentiation and natural death.

The so-called autocrine means that the substances secreted by oneself in turn act on oneself.

Looking to the future, XZ-C4 may become an induction therapy for cancer cell differentiation.

4). <u>XZ-C4 can inhibit cancer progression and metastasis</u>

<u>In the process of proliferation, cancer cells acquire the malignant nature of infiltration and metastasis. This phenomenon is called progression of malignancy.</u>

In order to research on cancer progression it is to require reproducible animal models. Therefore, the regressive cancer cell QR-32 isolated from mouse fibrosarcoma was made into this reproducible model. That is as the following:

a. Even if QR-32 is implanted subcutaneously in mice, it will not proliferate, but will completely disappear on its own; if it is injected into a human vein, there will be no metastatic nodules in the lung.

b. however, if gelatin sponge, which is a foreign body in the body, and QR-32 are transplanted under the skin of human mice, QR-32 will become proliferative cancer cell QRSP in vivo.

c. If QRSP is cultured in vitro and then transplanted into other mice, tumors will be proliferated even if there is no foreign body. If administered intravenously, lung metastasis will occur.

Using this model, we investigated whether XZ-C4 can affect cancer progression. The progress of this model is divided into two processes, namely:

a. The process of QR-32 transforming into proliferative cancer cell QRSP (pre-stage progression)

b. and QRSP proliferation into cancer (post-stage progression).

After being fed XZ-C4, the disease progression of the two types of model mice was inhibited, especially the most significant inhibition of the previous progress, and it was dependent on the dosage.

In terms of prolonging the survival time of the model mice, the QR-32 and gelatin sponge transplanted models all died within 65 days, while 30% of the XZ-C4 mice survived 150 days after tumor transplantation.

Previous experiments and clinical studies believe that XZ-C4 can enhance the immune effect and reduce the quinoa effect of anticancer drugs.

This experimental study proved that XZ-C4 has the effect of inhibiting the progression of cancer and can inhibit its invasion and metastasis.

5). XZ-C1+XZ-C4 immune regulation and control anti-cancer Chinese medicine

XZ-C1+XZ-C4 immune regulation anti-cancer Chinese medicine has the following characteristics as shown in Figure 1.

(1) Comprehensively improve the quality of life of patients with advanced cancer.

(2) Protect the thymus and improve immunity, protect the bone marrow, enhance hematopoietic function, improve immunity and control ability.

(3) Enhance physical fitness, relieve pain and improve appetite.

(4) Enhance the treatment effect and reduce the side effects of chemical therapy (Figure 1)

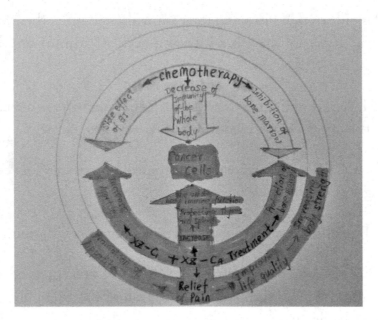

Figure 1 The characteristics of XZ-C immune regulation and control anti-cancer Chinese medicine

5. XZ-C immune regulation and control anti-cancer Chinese medicine is the result of the modernization of traditional Chinese medicine

XZ-C immune regulation and control anti-cancer Chinese medicine is not an empirical prescription, nor a famous old Chinese medicine prescription, but a scientific research result of the combination of Chinese and Western medicine and the modernization of traditional Chinese medicine.

It uses modern medical methods, experimental tumor experimental research methods, and modern pharmacology and medicine. Combining effectiveness research methods, after 7 years, more than 6000 cancer-bearing animal models:

200 kinds of commonly used so-called anti-cancer Chinese herbal medicines were screened in batches for animal experiments.

In vitro and in vivo tumor-bearing animals were screened by taste, and 48 kinds of Chinese medicines with good anti-cancer effects were screened out. Then these 48 kinds of natural medicines are formed into XZ-C1-10, and according to the respiratory system, digestive system, urinary system, gynecology, endocrine system, it was to make the animal models for each system such as liver cancer, gastric cancer, intestinal cancer, breast cancer, kidney bladder cancer, lung cancer and other cancer-bearing systems etc. to conduct in vivo pharmacodynamic experiments and toxicological experiments in tumor-bearing animals, then it was to make into XZ-C_1, XZ-C_2, XZ-C_3, XZ-C_4, XZ-C_5, XZ-C_6, XZ-C_7, XZ-C_8,,,,,, and other series of immune regulation anti-cancer Chinese medicines.

The material basis for traditional prescriptions to exert their unique curative effect in clinic is the chemical components.

Changes in the quality and quantity of chemical components directly affect the clinical efficacy of prescriptions.

Therefore, only by studying the changes in the quality and quantity of the chemical components in the prescriptions, clarifying the main effective ingredients of the preparations, and exploring the mystery of its unique curative effect from the perspective of molecular immunology, can the research on traditional prescriptions reach a new level.

The XZ-C immune regulating and Chinese medicine preparation is an innovation and reform of Chinese medicine preparations. It is not a compound liquid of mixed decoction, but a granular concentrate or powder of each medicine. Each crude medicine in each medicine still maintains its original ingredients. The function, molecular weight, and structural formula remain unchanged. It is made by modern scientific methods, not compounding. It keeps the original ingredients and functions of each flavor unchanged, which is convenient for evaluation and affirms the role and curative effect of the medicine.

15

The BRM-like effect and curative effect of XZ-C immune regulation and control anticancer Chinese medicine

Biological response modifiers (BRM) have opened up a new field of tumor biotherapy. At present, BRM as the fourth program of tumor treatment has received extensive attention from the medical community.

1). The Theory of Biological Response Regulation (BRM)

In 1982, Oldham founded the biological response modifier (BRM), or BRM theory, on this basis, in 1984, the family proposed **the fourth modality of cancer treatment -biological treatment.**

According to the BRM theory, under normal circumstances, the tumor and the body's defense are in a dynamic balance. The occurrence, invasion, and metastasis of tumors are completely caused by the imbalance of this dynamic balance. If the disordered state is artificially adjusted to a normal level, the growth of the tumor can be controlled and its regression can be achieved.

Specifically, BRM includes the following anti-tumor mechanisms:

1. *It is **to promote the enhancement** of the effect of the host's defense mechanism, or reduce the immunosuppression of the tumor-bearing host to achieve the ability of immune response to cancer.*

2. *It is **to administer natural or genetically recombined biologically active substances to enhance the host's defense** mechanism.*

3. *It is **to modify tumor cells** to induce strong host response.*

4. *It is to promote the differentiation and maturation of tumor cells and make them normalized.*

5. *It is to reduce the side effects of cancer chemotherapy and radiotherapy, and enhance the tolerance of the host.*

Biological therapy is to adjust this biological response by supplementing, inducing or activating the biologically active cell (or) factor with cytotoxic activity of the inherent BRM system in the body from outside.

Biological therapy is different from the other three treatment modes in the past, namely surgery, radiotherapy and chemical therapy, which target the tumor directly.

The scope of biological therapy obviously surpasses the traditional concept of immunotherapy.

This is because the dynamic balance between the body and tumor is not limited to immune response, but also involves various regulatory genes and cytokines related to tumor proliferation.

Tumor biotherapy mainly includes:

1. *Adoptive infusion of immunocompetent cells.*

2. *Production and application of lymphokines/cytokines.*

3. *Specific autoimmunity, including the application of tumor vaccines, monoclonal antibodies and cross-linked substances.*

The cells and humoral factors of the body's immune system are under **subtle regulation and control.** When they are out of balance (imbalance), the body's response or response ability will be **significantly** affected. The use of biological response modifiers is to restore the body state that is out of balance to normal balanced state to achieve the purpose of preventing and treating tumors.

Biological response modifiers regulate **the body's immune function and restore the suppressed body's immune system. The mechanism of action of these drugs is to activate the body's immune system to exert its regulatory function.** Many of them are derived from microorganisms and plants. Previously, these drugs were called immune enhancers, immune stimulants or immunomodulators.

Now they are collectively named as biological response modifiers BRM.

In recent years, some drugs with BRM-like effects have been discovered from Chinese medicine resources, and gratifying results have been achieved in experimental research and clinical applications.

2). The Biological response modifier

1)). Cytokines

a. It is produced by immune effector cells and related cells;

b. It is a cell regulatory protein with important biological activity and plays an important role in mediating a variety of immune responses in the body.

According to its biological activity, it can be divided into:

(1) Interleukin IL-2 is an interaction molecule between immune cells, which can promote the proliferation of activated T and B cells and activate the functions of killer cells such as NK cells.

(2) Interferon (IFN) has three types: IFN-a, IFN-Ý, and JFN-ß, which are a group of glycoprotein molecules.

(3) Colony stimulating factor (CSF) is a type of factor that stimulates the growth and differentiation of various types of hematopoietic stem cells.

It is divided into multidirectional CSF, granulocyte-macrophage CSF (GM-CSF), macrophage CSF (M-CSF) and granulocyte CSF (G-CSF).

(4) Tumor Necrosis Factor (TNF)

2)). Adoptive transfer of live immune cells

So far, there are 4 kinds of immune living cells used for tumor treatment:

(1). *Lymphokine killer cells (LAK).*

(2). *Tumor infiltrating lymphocytes (TIL).*

(3). *PWH-LAK and OKT-LAK:*

That is, PBL or TIL stimulated by Pokeweed (PWH) or immobilized anti-CD3 antibody (OKT3), both of which can increase the proliferation activity of LAK.

(4). *CD8 + CTL cells that recognize MHC I tumor antigens have strong tumor killing activity.*

3)). Tumor molecular vaccine

The current research on tumor vaccines mainly includes:

The unique vaccine against human tumor monoclonal antibodies can simulate tumor antigens to stimulate the body to produce anti-tumor responses.

4)). Natural herbal medicine with BRM-like effect

XZ-C immunomodulatory anti-cancer Chinese medicine has a BRM-like effect and curative effect.

3). The mechanism of action of biological response modifiers

BRM has the effect of regulating the host's immune response to tumors and killing tumor cells. Its mechanism of action is mainly expressed in the following five aspects:

1. It can directly regulate the growth and differentiation of cancer cells, and play a regulatory role in growth and differentiation.

2. It can enhance the sensitivity of cancer cells to the body's anti-cancer mechanism, which is beneficial to killing cancer cells.

3. It is to act on tumor blood vessels, affecting the nutrition and blood supply of the tumor, leading to tumor necrosis, while normal tissues are not damaged.

4. It is to stimulate the host's immune response against tumors.

5. It is to stimulate hematopoietic function, promote the recovery of bone marrow suppression, and enhance the tolerance to tumor treatment damage.

BRM can enhance the body's immune response and can strengthen the body's tumor immune surveillance.

<u>Its greatest effect occurs in patients with particularly small tumors. The effect is better when the cells are mutated or tumors are small, or with residual tumors or early tumors</u>.

Immunotherapy should be regarded as one of the comprehensive treatment measures for the treatment of malignant tumors.

Some people believe that immunotherapy can only deal with cancer cells below 10^5. If the cancer cells have formed obvious tumors, immunotherapy can **only play a role in restricting their growth**.

Although the immunotherapy has made great progress and has attracted the attention of the world, there are still different evaluations of the maturity of tumor immunotherapy. At present, it is considered to be a work worthy of in-depth research.

Its problems are:

(1). It is difficult to treat large tumors and can only be used as an auxiliary measure for surgery, chemotherapy and radiotherapy.

(2). Some tumor antigens only show individual specificity, so it is difficult to prepare anti-idiotypic antibodies.

<u>Several studies have shown that anti-tumor therapy does not require absolute specificity.</u>

Therefore, even if there is no specific antigen in the tumor, immunotherapy of tumor is still desirable.

The concentration of tumor-associated antigens expressed on malignant tumor cells is much higher than that of normal cells, and these differences are enough to make these antigens effective targets.

Moreover, because most tumor patients have weakened immune function, increased immunosuppressive factors in the body, and decreased production of IL-2, TNF and IFN, it is necessary to enhance the immune function of patients.

<u>In response to the above situation, how should we take countermeasures?</u>

a. *Because all cancer patients have low immune function, we should try to improve the patient's immunity during treatment.*

b. Due to the increase of immunosuppressive factors in tumor patients, we should deal with and antagonize them.

c. Since the production of IL-2, TNF and IFN in tumor patients is reduced, we should try to activate the increased production of these cytokines.

d. In order to further improve the effect of immunotherapy, it is necessary to further explore how to use the best combination with existing treatments.

4). Research overview of BRM-like immunomodulatory anticancer Chinese medicine

XZ-C immunomodulatory anti-cancer Chinese medicine has undergone 4 years of experimental research and 10 years of clinical verification to show that it has a BRM-like effect and curative effect, which is the drugs with similar BRM-like effects that are screened out from Chinese medicine resources.

XZ-C immunomodulatory anti-cancer Chinese medicine was selected by Professor XU ZE-China (XZ-C) in the laboratory from 200 kinds of Chinese herbal medicines.

First, the cancer cells were cultured in vitro, and 200 Chinese herbal medicines were screened in vitro one by one, and the experimental study on the direct damage of each drug to the cancer cells in the culture tube was observed. And it is to take the chemotherapy drug CTX and test tube cultured normal cells as the control group to compare the tumor inhibition rate.

As a result, a batch of drugs with inhibitory rate of cancer cell proliferation was selected.

Then, we will further create tumor-bearing animal models, and conduct experimental research on the in vivo tumor inhibition rate screening of tumor-bearing animal models for 200 kinds of Chinese herbal medicines, and conduct scientific, objective, and rigorous experimental screening, analysis, and evaluation.

The experiment proved that only 48 kinds of Chinese herbal medicines have good tumor inhibition rates, and the other 152 kinds of Chinese herbal medicines are common cancer treatment traditional Chinese medicines.

After this group of tumor-bearing experiments, the tumor inhibition rate in the tumor was screened, and it proved that there was no anti-cancer effect or the tumor inhibition rate was very low.

Our experimental screening work is mainly in vivo tumor suppression experiments in tumor-bearing animal models.

One experimental group of blindly traditional Chinese medicine observed chronic in vivo experiments for 3 months.

After 48 kinds of effective anti-cancer Chinese herbal medicines were screened out, each of the 2 and 3 crude drugs was combined to carry out in vivo tumor suppression experiments in tumor-bearing animals.

We also found that the anti-tumor effect of a single crude drug was not as good as the anti-tumor effect of the compound anti-tumor experiment of optimized combinations of several crude drugs.

It can be seen that the single crude drug only has an effect on the inhibition of tumor proliferation, and the optimized combination of multiple crude drugs not only inhibits the tumor proliferation of tumor-bearing mice, but also regulates the body, increases physical strength, increases immunity, and promotes the production of tumor suppressor cytokines, protect normal cells, promote anti-cancer factors, etc., have immune regulation effects.

Based on the in vitro experimental screening of single Chinese medicines in the early stage of 4 years in our laboratory and the in vivo anti-tumor experimental screening in tumor-bearing animal models, the combination was optimized through experiments and reorganized into $Z-_{Cl-10}$ immune control anti-pain after experiment, anti-metastasis, anti-relapse compound, and finally undergo clinical verification.

Since 1992, we have formed a collaborative group for clinical verification. So far, after 11 years of clinical verification and observation of more than 12,000 cancer patients in the oncology specialist outpatient clinic, they have achieved stable disease, improvement, improved symptoms, improved quality of life, and significantly extended survival.

Many patients with metastases stabilized their lesions without further spreading and metastasis. Some postoperative patients were unable to undergo radiotherapy or chemotherapy due to the decline in white blood cells and other reasons. Both have achieved good results.

5). The BRM-like effect and curative effect of XZ-C immunomodulatory anticancer Chinese medicine

Biological Response Modulation (BRM) was first described by Oldham in 1982 by the concept of BRM.

Its meaning is to adjust the body's ability to react or respond to external "attack" through biological response modifiers.

The cells and humoral factors of the body's immune system are under subtle or caressing regulation.

When the balance is out of balance, the body's response or response ability will be significantly affected.

The use of biological response modifiers is to restore the body state that is out of balance to a normal state of balance to achieve the purpose of preventing and treating diseases.

BRM has opened up a new field of tumor biotherapy.

At present, BRM, as the fourth mode of tumor treatment, has received extensive attention from the medical community.

Biological response modifiers regulate the immune function of the body and restore the function of the suppressed immune system.

The mechanism of action of these drugs is multifaceted, but no matter what the mechanism is, it exerts its regulatory function by activating the body's immune system.

Biological response modifiers, many of which are are derived from microorganisms and plants or may of which are from the *sources of microorganisms and plants, were previously called immune enhancers, immunostimulants, immune stimulants or immunomodulators, and are now collectively named as biological response modifiers or modifiers (BRM).*

XZ-C immunoregulatory anti-cancer and anti-metastasis Chinese medicines with good tumor inhibition rate through in vivo experiments in tumor-bearing mice in the laboratory screened out by the author can improve immunity, protect the thymus of the central immune organ, improve cellular immunity, protect thymus tissue function, improve immunity, protect bone marrow hematopoietic function, increase the number of red blood cells and white blood cells, activate immune cytokines, and improve immune surveillance in the blood.

The main pharmacological effect of XZ-C immune regulation Chinese medicine is anti-cancer and immune function promotion.

After 4 years of animal experiments, this group has screened out 48 kinds of medicines with high tumor inhibition rate, and it was to detect out 26 kinds of them by immunological and cytokine levels, which can enhance phagocytic function; or enhance cellular immunity; or enhance humoral immunity; or increase thymus weight; or promote bone marrow cell proliferation; or enhance T cell function; or enhance LAK cell activity; or enhance interferon IFN activity level; or enhance TNF activity; or enhance CSF colony stimulating factor; or inhibit platelet coagulation and inhibit thrombosis formation; or anti-tumor, anti-metastasis; or scavenging free radicals.

The anti-cancer mechanism of the above-mentioned XZ-C immunoregulatory anti-cancer Chinese medicine is:

1). It is to activate the body's **immune cell system**, promote the enhancement of the effect of the host's defense mechanism, and achieve the ability of immune response to cancer.

2). It is to activate the immune **cytokine system of** the body's anti-cancer mechanism, enhance the host's immune defense mechanism and improve the immune surveillance of immune cells in the body's blood circulation system.

3). It is to protect Thymus, promote immunity, that is, protects the thymus, increases immunity, protects blood production, protects the function of bone marrow growth, and stimulates bone hematopoietic function, promotes the recovery of bone marrow suppression, increases white blood cells, red blood cells, etc.

4). It is to reduce the side effects of radiotherapy and chemotherapy, and enhance the tolerance of the host.

5). The progression of cancer is caused by the imbalance between the biological characteristics of cancer cells and the body's ability to control cancer.

XZ-C immune regulation is to improve immunity and restore balance between the two.

6). It can directly regulate the growth and differentiation of tumor cells, and play a regulatory role in growth and differentiation.

7). It can increase the weight of the thymus so that the thymus does not shrink progressively, because the thymus glands progressively shrink when the cancer progresses.

8). It is to stimulate the host's anti-tumor immune response, enhance the anti-tumor ability of the machine, strengthen the sensitivity of cancer cells to the body's anti-cancer mechanism, and help kill cancer cells that are on the way to metastasis.

XZ-C immunomodulation Chinese medicine treatment of tumors can enable the host to produce a strong immune response to cancer cells, achieving the purpose of treating cancer.

XZ-C immune regulation and control anti-cancer Chinese medicine can cause the following immunological reactions in the host:

a. *It is to enhance, regulate or restore the host's immune response to tumors;*

b. *It is to stimulate the body's inherent immune function,*

c. *It is to activate the host's immune defense system;*

d. *It is to restore immune function.*

As mentioned above, the mechanism of action of XZ-C immunomodulatory anti-cancer Chinese medicine is basically similar to that of BRM, and the same therapeutic effect of BRM can be obtained in clinical use.

6). **XZ-C immune regulation and control anti-cancer Chinese medicine clinical application principles and scope of application**

1. **The application principle of XZ-C immune-regulating-and-control Chinese medicine**

XZ-C immunomodulatory anti-cancer Chinese medicine with BRM and BRM-like effects can enhance the **body's immune response** and enhance **the body's tumor immune surveillance**. It is better when the cells are mutated or the tumor is small.

Through surgery or radiation therapy, drug therapy works best when the tumor is minimized.

For those who have lost the opportunity for surgery, are in poor physique, and cannot tolerate radiotherapy and chemotherapy, immunotherapy has a certain effect, which can relieve symptoms and prolong survival.

After radical tumor resection, in order to reduce recurrence and metastasis, XZ-C immunomodulatory Chinese medicine treatment is feasible.

After surgical removal of larger tumors, in order to eliminate the remaining cancer cells and the cancer cells that may spread in the distance, XZ-C Immune regulation and control chinese medicine treatment is also feasible.

If the tumor cannot be removed, radiotherapy or chemotherapy can be used first to kill the tumor cells in large quantities and reduce the tumor load in the body, and then it is to use XZ-C immunoregulatory Chinese medicine treatment.

2. **Clinical observation and scope of application of XZ-C immune regulation and control Chinese medicine**

1). Anti-cancer postoperative metastasis:

It is to restore and improve postoperative immunity, improve postoperative quality of life, kill residual cancer cells after surgery, prevent metastasis, inhibit cancer cell proliferation, prevent recurrence, consolidate and enhance long-term efficacy.

Adaptation:

a. After radical resection of various advanced cancers;

b. After palliative resection of various cancers;

c. After the advanced cancerous wood that cannot be removed by exploration;

d. Only after gastrointestinal anastomosis or colostomy;

e. Those whose advanced cancer cannot be removed and have lost the indication for surgery;

f. After tumor resection + intubation drug pump.

2). It is to comprehensively improve the quality of life of patients with advanced cancer, prolong survival, inhibit cancer cell mitosis, control cancer cell proliferation, and improve overall immunity. The main objective is to resist spread and metastasis.

Adaptation:

(1) The short-term or long-term metastasis or recurrence after various tumors;

(2) Liver metastasis, lung metastasis, brain metastasis of various advanced cancers, or combined with cancerous pleural effusion and cancerous ascites.

(3) It is to relieve cancer pain:

Oral or external application of XZ-C drugs is used to treat various kinds of intractable pain and soften and reduce body surface transfer masses in advanced cancer.

(4) It is to cooperate with intermediary therapy or drug pump therapy to protect the liver, kidney, bone marrow hematopoietic system, thymus and other immune organs, improve immunity, metastasis.

Improve the overall immune status after drug injection, maintain, consolidate and enhance the intermittent and long-term efficacy of the injection (promote the curative effects of tumor treatment during the intermittent period and long-term), prevent metastasis, prevent spread, prevent recurrence, and comprehensively promote and improve the quality of life of patients with liver cancer after intermediary or intubation therapy, and prolong the survival period.

(5) While it is combined with radiotherapy and chemotherapy, it can reduce toxic and side effects, enhance the therapeutic effect, protect the liver, kidney, bone marrow hematopoietic system and immune organs, improve immune function, and promote white blood cells.

(6) XZ-C immunoregulatory anti-cancer Chinese medicine is used to combine with Chinese medicine decoction, such as:

a. It is used for the combination of Anticancer Shugan Xiaoshui Decoction for the treatment of liver cancer with ascites or metastatic cancerous ascites in the abdominal cavity;

b. It is to combine with Tuihuang Decoction to treat liver cancer and jaundice;

c. It is to combine with Jiangmei Zhuanyin Decoction to treat liver cancer with high transaminase and HbsAg positive.

d. It is to combine with Shengxuetang to treat leukopenia caused by chemotherapy.

3). *Application timing of XZ-C immune regulation and control anti-cancer Chinese medicine*

Cancer patients are mostly immunocompromised and should be treated immediately after diagnosis. The three major therapies of surgery, radiotherapy, and chemotherapy may further reduce the patient's immune function, which will reduce the patient's endurance to surgery, chemotherapy, and radiotherapy. And it reduces the immune surveillance in the immune cell system of the patient's body.

Therefore, immunotherapy should be started during surgery or during radiotherapy and chemotherapy.

XZ-C immunomodulatory Chinese medicines are all oral drugs. As long as patients can eat and drink, they can take XZ-C Chinese medicine.

a. It is generally to start taking the medication 1-2 weeks after surgery.

b. Before radiotherapy, chemotherapy, and during the interval between radiotherapy and chemotherapy, and after radiotherapy and chemotherapy, it is to continue to take XZ-C immunoregulatory Chinese medicine for a period of time, which may help reduce or control recurrence and metastasis.

This will help

a. *reduce the side effects of radiotherapy and chemotherapy.*

b. *prevent chemotherapy from causing weakened immune function and improve immunity,*

c. **promote the function of bone marrow blood production, protect the blood of the marrow,**

d. **activate the body's immune cell system and immune cytokine system, improve immune surveillance, and help prevent recurrence and metastasis.**

16

Typical cases of XZ-C immunomodulatory Chinese medicine in the treatment of malignant tumors

There are the following typical cases of which XZ-C immune modulation anti-cancer and anti-metastatic treatment were applied for various kinds of cancers and metastatic and relapsed patients, who were diagnosed and treated in our Hubei Group Medical Department and Shuguang Oncology Specialty Clinic of our National Collaborative Group on Anti-Cancer Research Combined with Chinese and Western Medicine:

1. **Typical cases of that the patient, who cannot have surgery, radiotherapy, or chemotherapy, only took XZ-C immune modulation anti-cancer chinese medicine to treat the cancer more than 5 years**

Case 1

Di XX, Male, 68 years old, Changzhou(hometown), Cadre(profession)
Medical record number xxxx

Diagnosis

Right upper lung central type lung cancer with left lung metastasis

The figure of the diagnosis and treatment of lung cancer cases as the following:

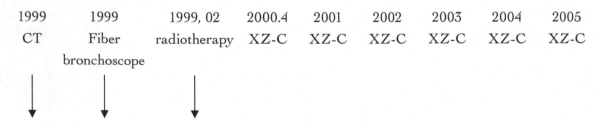

1999	1999	1999, 02	2000.4	2001	2002	2003	2004	2005
CT	Fiber bronchoscope	radiotherapy	XZ-C	XZ-C	XZ-C	XZ-C	XZ-C	XZ-C

Lung adenocarcinoma

Lung Cancer

XZ-C1+4+7

Medical history and treatment

The patients had coughed for 2 weeks in October 1998, with right shoulder pain, and treated with inflammation.

By January 1999, the cough had worsened, anorexia, fatigue, and weight loss gradually. CT was performed, and a mass was seen in the upper right hilar area, which was a central type of lung cancer.

In the Second Affiliated Hospital of Hubei Medical College, a fiberoptic bronchoscopy biopsy was done, the pathological report was lung adenocarcinoma. Neither the patient nor his family agreed to the operation.

In February 1999, a course of radiotherapy was performed. The side effects were so severe that the patient could not stick to radiotherapy.

At this time, the reexamination revealed two lesions in the left lung, which were metastases to the left lung, the patient coughs and has lots of sputum, blood in the sputum, and while walking, the patient has shortness of breath.

On April 23, 2000, the patient came to Shuguang Cancer Specialty Clinic for the treatment of XZ-C immunomodulatory anti-cancer Chinese medicine, taking XZ-C1 + X Z-C4 + XZ-C7, LMS + MDZ, after taking the medicine for 3 months, the patient felt symptoms better, spirit and appetite improve. By December 2000, his condition was stable, his spirit and appetite were good, his breathing was smooth, his complexion was ruddy, he walked like normal people, and sometimes he coughed.

The patient has long insisted on taking XZ-C1 + XZ-C4 + XZ-C7 daily for more than 4 years without interruption. It has been 5 years so far. He is in good health and walking activities are like normal healthy elderly. It is to see the picture below for the onset and treatment.

Analysis and evaluation

This patient is a right upper lung central type lung cancer.

In April 2000, he came to the specialist outpatient department with XZ-C$_{1+4+7}$ immunomodulatory therapy.

XZ-C1 can kill cancer cells and not normal cells;

XZ-C4 can improve immunity, promote thymus hyperplasia, increase immunity, protect bone marrow to produce blood;

XZ-C7 inhibits lung cancer cells, protects lung function, and reduces phlegm and inhibits cough.

Short-term radiotherapy is followed by long-term use of XZ-C immunomodulatory drugs to consolidate and enhance long-term efficacy.

XZ-C immunomodulatory drugs improve overall immune function, improve mental, appetite, and sleep, help the body's ability to resist disease and organ function, and restore nutrition and metabolism to help restore the patient's health.

This patient did not undergo surgery, and received radiotherapy in February 1999, and left lung metastasis occurred after radiotherapy, at our specialist clinic, the patients has long-term use of XZ-C immunomodulated anti-cancer and anti-metastasis Chinese medicine treatment, and has been insisting on long-term daily use of XZ-C medicine for more than 4 years, has never stopped, and achieved satisfactory results.

He has recovered well without any symptoms for 7 years. He came to the outpatient clinic in May 2005. He is generally in good condition, with good spirit and appetite, without any symptoms. Walking, activities, talking and laughing are like normal healthy elderly.

Case 2

Huang xx, female, 68 years old, from Hanyang of Wuhan
Medical record number XXXX

Diagnosis

Poorly differentiated squamous cell carcinoma of the lower esophagus

The Figure of the course of diagnosis and treatment of esophageal cancer as the following:

December 2000	January, 2001	2002	2003	2004	2005
Barium	XZ-C	XZ-C	XZ-C	XZ-C	XZ-C
Gastroscope					

Low differentiated esophageal
squamous cell carcinoma

XZ-C 1+2+3

Medical history and treatment

Vomiting began in December 2000, progressive dysphagia, eating obstruction, only semi-liquid food.

The esophago-endoscopy showed:

The esophageal stenosis, congestion, erosion, small ulcers, biopsy pathological report for poorly differentiated esophageal cancer of the lower esophagus.

Surgical treatment should be considered according to the condition, but due to economic difficulties, it is not possible to operate.

Therefore, the patient come to Shuguang Specialty Clinic for treatment of XZ-C immunomodulatory anti-cancer traditional Chinese medicine XZ-C1 + XZ-C4 + XZ-C2 integrated Chinese and Western medicine. After taking the medicine for 1 month, his spirit and appetite improved, and he consciously ate better, and he could eat vermicelli and porridge.

Then, patient stops to take XZ-C2 + XZ-C1 + XZ-C4 for 6 months. With good energy and appetite, you can eat soft rice, noodles and porridge. The patient continues to take the XZ-C immunomodulatory anti-cancer Chinese medicine XZ-C1 + XZ-C4 + XZ-C2. By June 2003, the patient had been taking the XZ-C medicine for 2 and a half years. The general condition and mental appetite were good. The patient can eat rice without discomfort and eat like normal people. He stopped the medicine for 4 and a half months,

Until October 16, 2003, after eating fried noodles, fried dough sticks, suddenly caused obstruction, vomiting color, cannot eat for 3 days, after fluid replacement support therapy improved, then continue to take XZ-$_{C1+4+2}$ to October 31st 2003, he resumed general diet and did not stop taking drugs.

He was revisited in May 2005. He is 71 years old this year. He is the same as the health elderly. The general condition is good, the mental appetite is good, and she has been able to eat general diet without discomfort. Living on the 7th floor, you can go downstairs every day, and sometimes you can do the job of pumping up the bicycle. The incidence and treatment process are shown in the figure below.

Analysis and evaluation

This patient is a poorly differentiated transient cell carcinoma of the lower esophagus. Diagnosed by gastroscopy and biopsy pathological section, he can only get liquid food and a small amount of semi-liquid food when he comes to the hospital. Due to financial difficulties, surgery, radiotherapy, or chemotherapy cannot be performed. The patient took XZ-C traditional Chinese medicine for immunoregulation for a long time without other treatment. After taking the medicine for half a year, the symptoms improved significantly. After taking the medicine for 2 and a half years, the patient completely recovered as normal healthy people. There was no discomfort when he took ordinary food. He was asked to review the barium meal, but he was unwilling to do it for economic reasons. In the past year, eating, living and normal health are as uncomfortable. It has been 5 years so far and is in good condition.

Long-term use of XZ-C immunomodulatory anti-cancer Chinese medicine can improve the patient's overall immunity, improve the patient's spirit and sleep.

XZ-C can protect the marrow and blood, protect the chest and increase immunity, promote the improvement of nutrition and metabolism, and eliminate free radicals, which is beneficial to the control and repair of lesions.

Case 3

Huang xx, female, 65 years old, Hubei, yellow people, farmers.
Medical record number XXXX

Diagnosis

<u>Mid-esophagus Cancer</u>
The figure of diagnosis and treatment of mid-esophageal cancer as the following:

2001 April	2001 June	2001 June	2002 June	2003 June $ZX\text{-}C_{4+2}$	2004 XZ-C	2005 XZ-C
	barium					
Onset of the disease	esophagus	$ZX\text{-}C_{1+4+2}$	XZ-C	XZ-C		

Medical history and treatment

Swallowing obstruction began in April 2001, and the chest and back swelling pain and discomfort gradually increased, and by June he could only enter liquid food and spit mucus.

On June 6, 2001, at the Peking Union Medical College Barium Meal Examination, there was a stenosis of about 10 cm in length 2 cm below the aortic arch, and a light arc-shaped filling defect of about 6 cm in length was seen on the left wall, mucosal interruption and destruction. Because of the economical situation, the surgery and radiotherapy and chemotherapy cannot be done, then On June 25th, 2001 the patient came to Shungguang outpatient center of oncology specialty for treatment of ZX-C $_{1+4+2}$. After 3 month of taking the medication, the general condition of this patient is good and spirit and appetite are good and the difficulty of swallowing are improved and can eat rice soup, noodle, and continue to take the $ZX\text{-}C_{1+4+2}$ medication until March, 2002, gradually eat rice, the common food. The patient changed to XZ-C4 + 2 in July 2003, then the patient revisited in April 2005, the patient is generally in good condition and has good appetite. Long-term administration of XZ-C immunomodulatory drugs has been in place for 5 years. It is in good condition, can eat common food, and can do light housework. See above the figure.

Analysis and evaluation

This patient is a cancer of the middle esophagus, without surgical treatment, radiotherapy, or chemotherapy. XZ-C immunomodulatory anti-cancer Chinese medicine XZ-C1 + XZ-C4 + XZ-C2. It has been 4 years so far, no transfer has occurred, it has been controlled. The patient is recovering well, is currently able to eat common rice, without discomfort, and like other healthy elderly, and can do some housework. The patient is still taking XZ-C1 + 4 Chinese medicine.

Case 4

Liu X female, 65 years old, from Jianshi County of Hubei Province
Medical record number xxxxx

Diagnosis
Primary massive hepatocellular carcinoma

The figure of diagnosis and treatment of liver recovery cases as the following:

1995	1995	1995	1996	1997	1998	1999	2000	2001	2002	2003	2004	2005
7.4,	7.11,	11	XZ-C	XZ-C	XZ-C	XZ-C	XZ-C	XZ-C	XZ-C	XZ-C	XZ-C	XZ-C
	XZ-C	Intervened										
		once										

Primary

Massive   XZ-C1+4+2

liver cave

Medical history and treatment

Due to upper abdominal discomfort for half a month, CT was performed at Union Hospital on July 4, 1995. Examination report 6.7cmX 7.1cmX9crn space occupying lesion in right lobe of liver, diagnosed as primary liver cancer, unwilling to undergo surgery or chemotherapy. On July 11, 1995, he came to the outpatient clinic of the Chinese and Western anti-cancer cooperative group to take XZ-C treatment. After 2 months, his mental and appetite improved significantly, and his weight increased.

On September 20, 1995, the reexamination of the CT mass was smaller than before.

In November 1995, he was treated with one-time embolization, but no other treatment was used. It has been more than 6 years of long-term adherence to XZ-C traditional Chinese medicine, and it has been 10 years so far.

He is currently in good health. He was followed up in May 2005. The general condition is good and he is as healthy as normal elderly. See picture.

Analysis and evaluation

This patient was diagnosed with primary liver cancer by CT examination on July 4, 1995. He was treated with XZ-C Chinese medicine 1 week later, and the tumor was reported to shrink after 2 months. On November 21, 1995, he was embolized 1 time. Since then, I have been taking XZ-C traditional Chinese medicine for only 10 years. It is as healthy as ordinary people.

Tips for this example

Intervention + XZ-C immune Chinese medicine has a good effect on liver cancer. Intervention can embolize the blood supply of the cancer artery, and chemotherapy can kill part of the cancer cells.

Majority of the patients still have alive cancer cells inside of the capsule and under the capsule after TAE. Due to incomplete necrosis, the tumor soon acquired collateral circulation and continued to grow.

XZ-C immune regulation and control Chinese medicine can protect the thymus and enhance immunity, protect the marrow and blood, and improve the overall immune function. In addition, 85% of liver cancer patients are on the basis of liver cirrhosis. TACE's chemotherapeutic drugs have certain damages to the liver. XZ-C Chinese medicine can protect liver function.

With the combination of intervention + XZ-C immune traditional Chinese medicine, the comprehensive application can achieve both inhibition of tumors and protection of the host, that is, it is not only eliminates evil but also strengthens the body; it is eliminating pathogens and strengthening the body, thereby consolidating and maintaining long-term effects.

Case 5

Huang XX, 53 years old, male, from Wuhan City
Medical record number xxxxx

Diagnosis

Primary massive liver cancer, post-hepatitis cirrhosis, advanced schistosomiasis, portal hypertension

The figure of diagnosis and treatment of primary liver cancer as the following:

2000	2000	2001	2001	2001	2002	2003	2004	2005
September	10.	19	1.2	3.31	11. 12	1. 9		
Intervention①	Intervention②	Intervention③	Intervention④	Intervention⑤	XZ-C	XZ-C	XZ-C	XZ-C

Right liver

Lesion   Intervene   XZ-C

13. 6cm X 11.8cm

Medical history and treatment

In September 2000, due to anorexia and abdominal discomfort, the Finance and Trade Hospital had a CT examination:

Right liver 13. 6cmX 11. 8cm low-density round lesions,

On September 7th of the same year, I went to Xiehe Hospital for MRI examination:

A huge space-occupying lesion of 13.1cm X 11.4 cm X 12. S cm was seen in the right lobe of the liver.

Diagnosed at Union Hospital on September 13 as:

Massive liver cancer in the right lobe of the liver.

Do right hepatic artery infusion chemotherapy + embolization;

Performed the second hepatic artery chemoembolization on October 19, 2000;

Do it for the third time on January 2, 2001;

The fourth time was on March 30, 2001;

It was the fifth time on November 12, 2001.

Interventional chemotherapy drugs are HCPT 25mg + 5-FU 1000mg, lipiodol 10ml + MMC 10mg.

The current situation is generally good.

The lesion changes after intervention are as follows:

On October 12, 2000, CT examination of the right lobe of the liver lesion 11.1 cmX11.8 cm,

On December 4, 2000, CT examination of the right lobe of liver lesion 10.8cmX9.8cm.

The lesion is basically stable and has shrunk.

In February 2001, CT examination of the right lobe of the liver lesion 10. 5cmX9.5cm,

CT examination on September 3, 2001, the 9.8 cm X 8.9 cm lesion in the right lobe of the liver was basically stable and reduced.

On January 9, 2002, I came to Shuguang Oncology Specialty Clinic to take XZ-C immunomodulatory anti-cancer medicine XZ-C1+4+5. After taking the medicine, the general condition is good, and the spirit, appetite and sleep are good.

The patient comes to the outpatient clinic for follow-up visits every month to take XZ-C1+4+5 immune-regulating Chinese medicine. The condition of the follow-up visit on October 21, 2002 is stable, with good general condition, good spirits, appetite, urine and bowel as usual, normal walking activities, and good health recovery, B-ultrasound and CT review, the lesions are stable as before, do housework in the morning, play cards in the afternoon, live a regular life, exercise regularly, have never caught a cold, and have been 4 and a half years, just like healthy elderly people, with good quality of life without discomfort. See Figure above.

Analysis and Evaluation

This case is a primary massive liver cancer. After 5 interventional treatments, the cancer focus has been reduced and good results have been achieved. The last intervention was November 12, 2001. At this time, the right lobe lesion was 9.8 cmX8. 9cm, started to take XZ-C1+4+5 treatment at Shuguang Oncology Clinic on January 9, 2002, *XZ-C1 can kill cancer cells, but not normal cells; XZ-C4 protects the thymus, prevents thymic atrophy, High immunity, XZ-C5 protects the liver, and XZ-C Chinese medicine has been taken daily for 3 years. So far, it has been 4 and a half years. The general condition is good and the condition is stable, without metastasis or development. Good spirit and appetite, walking activities as usual.*

The treatment experience of this case is:

Interventional therapy is first used for massive liver cancer to shrink and stabilize the cancer focus, and then take XZ-C immunomodulatory Chinese medicine to consolidate the long-term effect, protect the liver, increase immunity, and control blood metastasis.

Case 6

Qi xx, male, 51 years old, cadre, from Yingcheng of Hubei.
Case number xxxxxx

Diagnosis

Primary liver cancer

The figure of diagnosis and treatment of primary liver cancer as the following:

1997	1997	1998	1999	1999. 11	2002	2002. 6
10. 30	11.25	XZ-C	XZ-C	XZ-C	XZ-C	
CT diagnosis	XZ-C$_{1+4+5}$					
B ultrasound				*Died after surgery in a foreign* hospital		

Confirmed liver cancer

Taking XZ-C1, XZ-C4, XZ-C5 Chinese medicine,
without radiotherapy or chemotherapy, basically recovered to health

Medical history and treatment

CT examination on October 30, 1997 found:

The left liver occupies a size of 4. 6cm X 3.6 cm, and the right lobe of the liver occupies a size of 1.6 cm X 1.6 cm. Report: Liver cancer.

Color Doppler ultrasound in Union Hospital on November 11, 1997:

The left lobe of the liver occupies the size of 5.9cm X 4.0 cm X 5.4 cm, and the right lobe of the liver occupies the size of 2.1cm X 1.8 cm. Hepatic angiography report: liver cancer. HB Ag (ten), AFP (one).

Due to poor liver function, he cannot be operated or intervened.

Aclohic

Alcohol Drinking history for 40 years, a meal of about 250ml, suffering from hepatitis B in 1996, schistosomiasis in 1966.

On November 25, 1997, I came to the Anti-Cancer Collaborative Group for the treatment of combined Chinese and Western medicine: XZ-Cl, XZ-C4,XZ-C5.

In 1998 and 1999, the patient came to Wuchang outpatient clinic from Yingcheng County for review and medicine by himself every month.

The patient is in good condition, ruddy, talking and laughing as usual.

After a follow-up visit on November 2, 1999, the liver B-ultrasound lesions were significantly reduced.

Can be engaged in light physical work without discomfort. For more than 2 years, I have been taking XZ-C1+4+5 without interruption. After consciously taking the medicine, I have good appetite and good physical strength.

At the beginning of June 2002, I was introduced to Beijing xx General Hospital for medical treatment. (Before I went to Beijing, my condition was generally good, and my walking activities were as usual).

In the hospital for surgical exploration, there was a liver cancer mass of about 5cm X 6cm during the operation, which was the same as the onset 5 years ago. There were tumor thrombi in the bile duct, no metastasis in the abdominal cavity, no ascites, no intrahepatic metastasis, but the tumor was close to the hepatic portal and difficult to remove, Is to take the bile duct tumor thrombus and put T tube drainage. After the operation, there was no urine, acute renal failure, and death 6 days after the operation. See Figure the above.

Analysis and Evaluation

CT of the patient found on October 30, 1997, the left liver 4. 6cmX3. 6cm occupying lesions;

On November 11, 1997, the right lobe of the liver was found to occupy 2.1cmX 1.8cm. Due to poor liver function, he could not be operated or intervened. No other treatment was used.

The $XZ\text{-}C_{1+4+5}$ immunomodulatory therapy has been used for more than 5 years in the outpatient clinic of the Anti-Cancer Cooperation Group on November 25, 1997, and he is in good health.

The treatment experience of this patient is: XZ-C Chinese medicine improves the overall immune function of the host (cellular and humoral immune function), protects the central and peripheral immune organs, protects the liver and kidney, induces tumor suppressor factors, stabilizes the cancer focus, and prevents metastasis and spread.

XZ-C Chinese medicine is a non-injury treatment. It can sincerely strengthen the body to eliminate evil. In addition, the patient's mental state is good, which is conducive to overcoming the disease and conducive to recovery, thus achieving better curative effects.

This patient has been taking XZ-C Chinese medicine for 5 years in a stable condition. The liver cancer has not increased or metastasized. He is generally in good condition and has no discomfort. He walks and talks and laughs as normal.

During my visit to Beijing for treatment this time, xx General Hospital was diagnosed with hepatocellular carcinoma by surgical exploration and pathology. The tumor was in the hilar of the liver and could not be removed. Because of the bile duct tumor thrombus, the tumor thrombus was taken and T tube drainage was performed. The patient has been anuria after the operation and died of acute renal failure. If the liver and kidney are not attacked by surgical exploration, this may not necessarily be the case. It is a pity!

2. **The tumor cannot be removed by surgical exploration, and radiotherapy or chemotherapy cannot be performed.**

Treat typical cases of more than 4 years with XZ-C immune regulation and control anti-cancer Chinese medicine

Case 1

Cheng xx, male, 64 years old, from Xinzhou, Hubei, cadre
Medical record number xxxxx

Diagnosis

Retroperitoneal tumor

The figure of retroperitoneal tumor diagnosis and treatment process as the following:

1999	1999	2000	2001	2002
March	April	XZ-Cl+4	XZ-Cl+4	XZ-Cl+4

Surgical exploration

XZ-Cl+4

Medical history and treatment

On January 6, 1999, there was sudden chest discomfort, pain, and vomiting. The emergency department considered it to be "acute gastroenteritis", the surgical consultation suspected pancreatitis, and the gastroscopy on March 3 showed duodenal obstruction.

Laparotomy on March 6, 1999 showed that the retroperitoneal tumor was encapsulating large blood vessels. During the operation, it was found that there was a mass of about 6cmX 9cm at the root of the small mesenteric. The transverse part of the duodenum is difficult to remove, but the proximal end of the duodenum is anastomosed with Roux-y of the jejunum.

The tumor cannot be removed, so a combination of Chinese and Western medicine is ordered.

On April 4, 1999, the patient came to Shuguang Oncology Specialty Clinic to start taking XZ-C1, XZ-C4 immunomodulatory anti-cancer Chinese medicine.

He started taking XZ-C1+4 Chinese medicine continuously from May 15, 1999 to February 2002. During this period, outpatient review and medicine were taken from time to time, and he was in good health. See Figure 17-70

Analysis and Evaluation

This patient was found to be a retroperitoneal tumor by laparotomy on March 6, 1999. The large blood vessels were tightly wrapped around the roots of the mesentery and could not be resected, and he did not dare to take slices or to have biopsy for further analysis. However, judging from its hard, fixed, and uneven surface, it should be a malignant tumor.

After taking XZ-C Chinese medicine for 4 years in the cancer specialist clinic, the condition is stable, has not developed or metastasized, and is still in good health.

Case 2

Fang xx, male, 50 years old, from Luotian, Hubei, farmer
Medical record number xxxxx

Diagnosis

After pancreatic head cancer exploration

The figure of diagnosis and treatment of pancreatic cancer as the following:

1996, November	1996 December	1998 XZ-C	1999 XZ-C	2000 XZ-C	2001 XZ-C

Surgical

Exploration

Pathological section   XZ-C1+4

Pancreatic cancer

Medical history and treatment

The patient had the upper abdominal discomfort for 3 months.

On November 23, 1996, he had a caesarean examination for jaundice in the local hospital:

During the operation, no stones were found in the biliary tract, and the pancreatic head was enlarged and could not be removed. The pathology of the sample was pancreatic cancer.

Postoperative CT diagnosis:

It is carcinoma of the head of the pancreas with dilatation of the bile duct in the liver.

The postoperative jaundice persisted, so I came to Shuguang Oncology Clinic to take XZ-C Chinese medicine for immunotherapy on December 11, 1996.

After taking the medicine for 1 month, the general condition improved, and the spirit and appetite improved.

When she was discharged from the hospital, she still had jaundice and excessive sweating. After continuing to take XZ-C medicine and Shugan Lidan Tuihuang Decoction for 2 months, the jaundice gradually subsided and the pain eased.

Four months later, the jaundice disappeared, the spirit was good, the appetite was good, and the abdomen still had slight pain.

By July 1998, he resumed work, participated in light labor, and his face was full of red light. In the past few years, he continued to take XZ-C Chinese medicine, and his health was restored.

On April 6, 2004, the patient's family brought another patient to this outpatient clinic to get sick. He said that Fang xx old man: In good health, he walks frequently, can do housework, and is in harmony with normal healthy old people. See Figure as the above.

Analysis and Evaluation

This patient had pancreatic head cancer and jaundice. He was unresectable by laparotomy on November 28, 1996.

Postoperative diagnosis: pancreatic head cancer with intrahepatic bile duct dilatation.

The patient came to the clinic on December 11, 1996. After taking XZ-C immune regulation anti-cancer Chinese medicine and Shugan Lidan Tuihuang Decoction for a long time, the jaundice gradually subsided after 7 months.

It was to continue to take XZ-C daily for a long time to increase immunity until The patient recovered well in July 1998. ***Taking XZ-C immune regulation and control anti-cancer Chinese medicine can soothe the liver and promote gallbladder, strengthen the body, promote blood circulation and remove blood stasis.***

He continued to take the medicine for more than 4 years, and then changed to intermittent medicine to maintain the effect, so far for 9 years, the patient's health condition is still good.

Case 3

Li xx, male, 53 years old, from Caidian, Wuhan, farmer
Medical record number xxxxx

Diagnosis

Primary massive liver cancer, advanced schistosomiasis cirrhosis.

The figure of the massive primary liver cancer as the following:

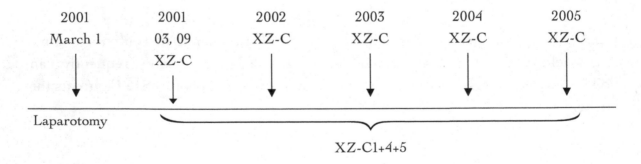

Medical history and treatment

On January 22, 2001, he felt pain in his right back and back.

On February 26, a B-ultrasound examination revealed a lump in the liver.

On January 31, 2001, CT showed a 14cmX 11cm space-occupying lesion in the right lobe of the liver, which was diagnosed as massive liver cancer in the right lobe.

An exploratory laparotomy was performed at Tongji Hospital on March 1. The tumor was too large to be resected, and a drug pump was placed in the portal vein.

After the operation, the drug pump was injected once (mitomycin and 5-FU).

The patient has a history of schistosomiasis for 30 years.

On March 9, 2001, he came to Shuguang Oncology Specialty Clinic to take XZ-C immunoregulatory Chinese medicine treatment.

It was to use XZ-C1+4+5, LMS, MDZ internally or orally and use XZ-C3 for external application.

After taking the medicine for 1 month, the general condition improved, the spirit and appetite improved, and the mass under the costal margin of the right upper abdomen became soft and shrunk.

After taking the medicine for 3 months, the general condition is good, the appetite and sleep are good, the physical strength is gradually restored, and the walking activities are as normal.

Re-examination of B-ultrasound on October 22, 2001:

See 6cmX 7.8cm occupancy on the right lobe of liver, continue to take XZ-C1+4+5 treatment and XZ-C3 external application,

On November 19, 2003, a comprehensive review showed that the intrahepatic lesions in B-ultrasound were the same as before, the kidneys were not abnormal, the chest radiographs were not abnormal, the subclavian lymph nodes were not palpable, and the right subclavian mass was significantly reduced, soft, with clear borders. There was no pain, continue to take XZ-C1+4+5, see Figure of the above.

Analysis and Evaluation

This patient had a massive liver cancer, which could not be removed by surgical exploration, and was given 1 chemotherapy session with a drug pump in the portal vein.

In March 2001, he started to come to the clinic to take the Chinese medicine XZ-C1+4+5 for immune regulation and anticancer and XZ-C3 for external application. The medication has been persisted for 4 years. The condition is stable, no further development, and no metastasis.

Case 4

Ke xx, male, 54 years old, Hubei Yangxin, cadre
Medical record number xxxxx

Diagnosis

Primary liver cancer

The figure of Primary liver cancer diagnosed and treated as the following:

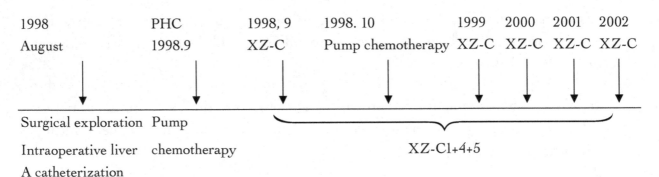

1998		PHC	1998, 9	1998. 10		1999	2000	2001	2002
August		1998.9	XZ-C	Pump chemotherapy		XZ-C	XZ-C	XZ-C	XZ-C

Surgical exploration Pump

Intraoperative liver chemotherapy

A catheterization

XZ-C1+4+5

Medical history and treatment

Her right upper abdomen was painful for half a month and her appetite lost. CT examination at Yangxin County Hospital found that the right anterior lobe, right posterior lobe, and left inner lobe occupied lesions. Diagnose primary liver cancer.

Laparotomy was performed on August 20, 1998. During the operation, the main tumor was found at the hilar of the liver. Both left and right livers had metastases and could not be resected. A chemotherapy pump was used in the hepatic artery.

A chemotherapy pump could be placed in the hepatic artery. Second, cisplatin + adriamycin was injected into the pump.

For the second chemotherapy in October 1998, carboplatin + adriamycin was injected through a pump.

The pump was not used again because it was blocked.

On September 8, 1998, he came to the outpatient clinic of the Anti-cancer Research Cooperation Group of Integrated Traditional Chinese and Western Medicine and was treated with the traditional Chinese medicine XZ-C1+4+5.

After taking the medicine for 1 month, I have good appetite, weight gain, ruddy complexion, a soft abdomen, liver and spleen are not in reach, general condition is good, and I am completely self-care. Every month I take a long-distance bus from Yangxin to Wuhan clinic for recheck and get medicine. The patient feels no discomfort, and there is no abnormality in the physical examination.

When he came to the clinic for follow-up visit on June 4, 2002, he was generally in good condition, with a ruddy complexion, walking, moving, talking and laughing like normal healthy people, and no abnormalities in the physical examination. See Figure as the abobe.

Analysis and Evaluation

CT of this patient found space-occupying lesions in the anterior lobe, posterior lobe, and left inner lobe of the liver.

On August 20, 1998, a laparotomy was performed.

The liver cancer had metastases in both the left and right livers and could not be resected. A chemotherapy pump was installed and chemotherapy was injected after the operation for twice. On September 8, 1998, XZ-C1+4+5 immunomodulation Chinese medicine was used in the outpatient clinic of the cooperative group. By the end of 2002, he was in good health. No distant metastasis occurred.

This example suggests that : when liver cancer cannot be resected through laparotomy, a chemotherapy pump can be placed in the hepatic artery, and XZ-C1+4+5 immunoregulatory Chinese medicine treatment can be used after the operation to protect the thymus, bone marrow, and liver, improve overall immune function, and induce the body to produce anti-cancer factors In order to control cancer foci, tumor development can be controlled.

A chemotherapy pump can be placed in the hepatic artery, a catheter can be placed in the liver during the surgical exploration, and chemotherapy through the pump

3. *Recurrence after radical resection, typical cases of more than 5-10 years treated with XZ-C immunomodulation anti-cancer Chinese medicine*

Case 1

Mao xx, male, 48 years old, from Tianmen, Hubei, cadre
Medical record number xxxxxx

Diagnosis

Primary liver cancer

The figure of diagnosis and treatment of primary liver cancer is as the following:

1994	1994	1994	1995	1996.12	1997	1998		2005
8 11	8.26	11.26	XZ-C	XZ-C	XZ-C	XZ-C	medication treating for 7 years	XZ-C
		XZ-C						

B ultrosond	Operation			
Find a tumor			XZ-C 1+4	

Medical history and treatment

On August 11, 1994, due to fatigue and fatigue, he went to the local county hospital for a B-ultrasound, and found a 4. lcmX4.5cm space-occupying lesion in the left liver.

On August 26, 1994, the left hepatic lobe was resectioned in Union Hospital. Pathological section: hepatocellular carcinoma, no other treatment.

After the operation, he came to the XZ-Cl+4+5 anti-cancer immune Chinese medicine treatment at the outpatient department of the Anti-cancer Cooperation Group of

Integrated Traditional Chinese and Western Medicine. After taking the medicine, he had good spirits, appetite, and physical recovery.

The patients have been taking XZ-C immune traditional Chinese medicine for a long time, and I come to the outpatient clinic for check-ups and medicines every month. I am generally in good condition and have resumed work.

By the B-ultrasound re-examination on December 14, 1996, it was found that there was a space-occupying lesion of about 1.3cmX 1.8cm in the left extrahepatic lobe. Resection of the left extrahepatic lobe was performed at Union Hospital on December 30, 1996. After the operation the patient continued to take XZ-C1+ 4+5 anti-relapse and anti-metastasis immune Chinese medicine treatment.

The patient insists on taking XZ-C Chinese medicine daily for a long time without interruption.

In May 2005, he returned to the clinic. The general condition was good, the complexion was ruddy, the body was as strong as an ordinary person, and he had resumed physical work for 11 years, and he had good spirits and appetite. The liver, gallbladder and pancreas B-ultrasound was reviewed, and no abnormalities were found. See Figure as the abobe.

Analyze and evaluate this case

On August 26, 1994, the patient underwent a left hepatic lobectomy due to a 4. lcmX4.5cm space-occupying lesion of the left liver, and was treated with XZ-C immunomodulatory Chinese medicine after surgery.

On December 30, 1996, it was found that the left liver had a space-occupying lesion of 1.3cmX1.8cm. The left lateral lobectomy was performed again. After the operation, XZ-C Chinese medicine treatment was performed. After long-term use of XZ-C1+4+5, he is still healthy. The condition is good, and it has been 11 years since he resumed physical work.

This example suggests:

After liver cancer resection, the patient takes XZ-C1+4+5 immunomodulatory Chinese medicine for a longer period of time, which protect the Thymus and increase immune function, protect bone marrow and promote blood, protect the liver function, improve the overall immune function and disease resistance, surgery + XZ-C immune Chinese medicine, can Consolidate the long-term effect after surgery.

Case 2

Cai xx, male, 65 years old, from Wuhan, cadre
Medical record number xxxxxx

Diagnosis

Gastric cardia cancer poorly differentiated adenocarcinoma, recurrence after radical resection, recurrence of remnant stomach cancer

The figure of diagnosis and treatment of recurrent cancer after radical gastric cancer as the following:

1993	1994	1996. 6 1997. 6 1998. 6 1999. 6 1999. 12 2000. 5 2001 2002 2003 2004
June	March	

Radical	Recurrent cancer
Surgery	of remnant stomach
for Gastric	
Cancer	

Medical history and treatment

The patient was diagnosed with gastric cancer due to epigastric pain for 1 year and underwent a radical subtotal gastrectomy at Union Hospital in June 1993.

After the operation, the FM regimen was given 1 chemotherapy. Due to anemia, the body was weak and could not be treated. The test was WBC1.9X10^9/L.

Eight months after the operation, pain under the xiphoid process accompanied by vomiting, pain in the left upper abdomen for half a year, went to the Xiehe Hospital barium meal on March 25, 1994; irregular filling defect at the upper end of the remnant stomach, partial membrane destruction, and anastomotic narrowing.

The conclusion of the barium meal is:

Recurrent cancer in the remnant stomach.

B-ultrasound on May 3, 1996:

No space-occupying lesions were seen in the liver. Because the patient cannot eat rice, he can eat semi-liquid food and noodles. The patient felt fatigue, weakness, poor spirits, and reluctance to operate again. Since 1996, the outpatient department of the Anti-cancer Cooperation Group of Integrated Traditional Chinese and Western Medicine has been treated with XZ-C series of immunological Chinese medicines.

After taking the medicine, the general condition of the patient improved, and the spirit and appetite improved. He has taken XZ-C medicine daily for more than 8 years. When I came to the follow-up consultation on March 6, 2004, the patient was generally in good condition, with a ruddy complexion, good spirits and appetite, talking and laughing. As usual, eat porridge and steamed bread without discomfort. See Figure as the above.

Analysis and Evaluation

This patient received a radical resection of gastric cancer in June 1993. In March 1994, cancer recurred in the remnant stomach and the anastomosis was narrow.

With XZ-C1+4, immune traditional Chinese medicine treatment, no other treatment, so far, 10 years and 2 months, recovered to health in good condition.

This example suggests

Recurrent cancer in the remnant stomach, and the anastomotic stoma is not completely obstructed, and you can still eat. After XZ-C1+4 immune traditional Chinese medicine treatment for Thymus protection and immune function improvement, it can control tumors, prevent metastasis, stabilize the lesions, make the condition improve significantly, and survive for a long time.

Case 3

Chen xx, male, 62 years old, from Wuhan, senior engineer
Medical record number xxxxx

Diagnosis

Right renal pelvis tumor, bladder cancer recurred after surgery

The figure of diagnosis and treatment of bladder cancer is as the following:

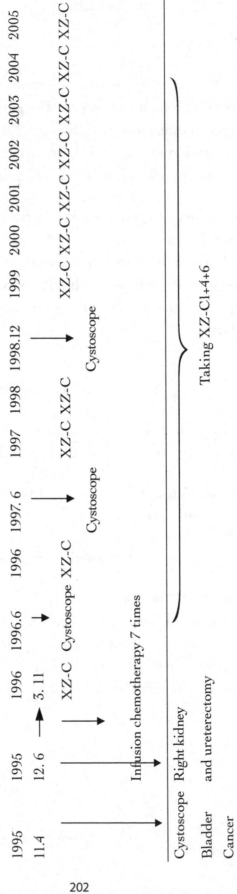

Medical history and treatment

The patient has hematuria for 2 years, had cystoscopy on November 4, 1995, which was diagnosed as bladder cancer. CT found a tumor of the right renal pelvis on November 21, 1995,

On December 6, 1995, he underwent right kidney and ureter resection, bladder sleeve resection, and the patient had 7 postoperative local infusion chemotherapy.

On March 8, 1996, the cystoscope was re-examined, and it was found that there was a rigid bulge on the left side of the bladder to prevent recurrence.

On March 11, 1996, I came to the cooperative group outpatient clinic with XZ-C1+4+6 immunomodulatory Chinese medicine alone. After taking the medicine, the patient's appetite improved.

The cystoscope was reviewed on June 24, 1996, the surface was smooth and the new organisms had disappeared. The patient continued to take XZ-C Chinese medicine for a long time.

As of June 11, 1997 and December 28, 1998, there were no abnormalities in the cystoscopy twice.

The follow-up visit on June 26, 1999 was in good condition. The patient has been taking Z-C1+4+6 daily for 10 years, which prevented the recurrence or metastasis of bladder tumors.

The patient returned on May 6, 2005, and the patient is in good condition and has fully recovered to a normal healthy elderly. See Figure 17-13,

Analysis and Evaluation

This patient had a recurrence of bladder cancer after surgery. He has been taking XZ-C immunoregulatory Chinese medicine for more than 10 years, preventing the recurrence or metastasis of bladder cancer. His condition is good. After repeated cystoscopy, he has completely returned to normal.

This example suggests:

XZ-C immune regulation Chinese medicine can improve the patient's immune function, promote cancer stability, and prevent the recurrence and metastasis of bladder cancer.

Case 4

Ling xx, male, 68 years old, from Wuhan, professor
Medical record number xxxxx

Diagnose

Recurrence of bladder cancer after surgery

The figure of diagnosis and treatment of bladder cancer recurrence after surgery as the following:

1994	1996	1999.5	1999.6	1999.7	2000.7	2001	2002	2003	2004	2005
surgery	surgery	intervention	intervention	XZ-C	XZ-C	Intervention				
						XZ-C	XZ-C	XZ-C	XZ-C	XZ-C

Bladder infusion Bladder infusion

Bladder   Recurrence Recurrence   Recurrence
cancer   on cystoscopy
Resection Resection   intervention

Medical history and treatment

In April 1994, he underwent bladder cancer resection at the Provincial People's Hospital. The disease was checked for transitional cell carcinoma.

After the operation, bladder perfusion chemotherapy MMC was stopped due to a significant decrease in white blood cells.

At the beginning of 1996, it was checked for recurrence, and 8 tumors in the bladder were removed again.

After the operation, the bladder was infused twice a month. After 3 months, the bladder was infused for 3 months. After 3 months, the bladder was infused for another 3 months, twice a month. It was done at the beginning of 1997 and in May 1998 in Concord The hospital cystoscopy had flocculation, and the B-ultrasound re-examination in December was cystitis.

In April 1999, he underwent cystoscopy due to hematuria. A 4cm2 tumor was found in the triangle area. CT and biopsy were all bladder cancer.

In March 1999, he received interventional bladder arterial chemotherapy perfusion.

In June for the second intervention 5-FU + MMC + carboplatin, the white blood cells dropped to 2X109/L after blood transfusion.

In September, I did the third intervention with 5-FU + MMC + L-camptothecin. The white blood cells dropped to 1.2 X 109/L, which was an injection of Gelifen Shengbai needle.

Past history:

In 1992, the stroke was over, high blood pressure (160/90mmHg), diabetes.

He suffered from hepatitis in 1984 and cirrhosis in 1998.

Family history: second brother (after hepatitis B) liver cancer, younger brother rectal cancer.

When I came to the clinic in July 1999 because of low blood picture after interventional treatment, I used Husui Shengxue Decoction and XZ-C1+4+6 Chinese medicine to promote anti-cancer. After taking the medicine for 6 months, the blood picture rose to normal, and my spirit and appetite were also improved. Significant improvement, continue to take the medicine.

In July 2000, cystoscopy showed that the bladder was filled well, and a 1.3cmX0.6cm medium echo light cluster was seen in the triangle area. Considering a recurrent tumor, I continued to take the medicine until June 2001. The patient had frequent urination due to prostate hyperplasia. CT review of bladder cancer lesions was larger than before (compared with February 1999), and bladder artery intervention was performed once. Continue to take XZ-C1+4+6 until the bladder CT was reviewed on July 6, 2002. The bladder cancer lesions were smaller than before. After taking the drug, the general condition was good, the appetite was good, and there was no hematuria. It has been 6 years and the lesion control is stable. No further development, no distant metastasis, see as the above Figure.

Analysis and Evaluation

This patient is a transitional cell carcinoma of the bladder. After resection, it has recurred many times. Long-term infusion chemotherapy failed to prevent the recurrence. Due to bladder perfusion and multiple cystoscopy for many years, as well as prostatic hyperplasia and urethra stricture, cystoscopy is difficult. Long-term use of XZ-C immune regulation anti-cancer medicine XZ-C1+ 4 + 6, bladder neoplasms have not developed, no metastasis, onset has been 11 years, the general condition is good, the spirit and appetite are both good, and sometimes hematuria appears when walking for a long time..

Case 5

Qi xx, female, 67 years old, from Shijiazhuang City, worker
Medical record number xxxxx

<u>Diagnosis</u>

<u>Abdominal myxoma recurred after surgery</u>

The figure of diagnosis and treatment of postoperative recurrence of abdominal myxoma is as the following:

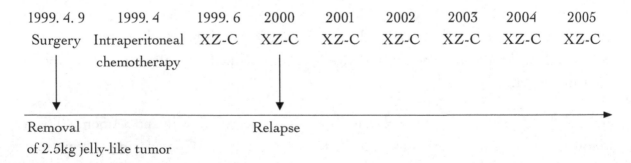

| 1999. 4. 9 | 1999. 4 | 1999. 6 | 2000 | 2001 | 2002 | 2003 | 2004 | 2005 |
| Surgery | Intraperitoneal chemotherapy | XZ-C | XZ-C | XZ-C | XZ-C | XZ-C | XZ-C | XZ-C |

Removal
of 2.5kg jelly-like tumor

Relapse

Medical history and treatment

In the past two years, the abdomen is getting bigger and ascites.

She was admitted to Tongji Hospital in March 1999, with ascites sign++, frog abdomen, palpable intra-abdominal mass, on April 9 laparotomy:

The abdominal cavity was filled with jelly-like masses of varying sizes, which were excised one by one, weighing 2.5 kg. 5-FU 500 mg was placed during the operation and chemotherapy was placed in the abdominal cavity.

From the 4th day after operation, 5-FU 500mg was injected once a day for 5 days and carboplatin 100mg once a day for 3 days.

Came to the Shuguang Oncology Clinic on June 16, 1999, and took XZ-C immunoregulatory anti-cancer Chinese medicine XZ-C1+4. After taking the medicine for 2 months, she had good spirits, appetite, and weight gain.

Physical examination:

The supraclavicular is not abnormal, the abdomen is flat and soft, and the abdomen is not abnormal, ascites (一), continue to take XZ-C immunoregulatory Chinese medicine for a long time, and come back to the clinic every month to get the medicine until November 26, 2000.

The upper middle abdomen can be deducted from the physical examination, and the mass of the fist of approximately adults is hard, with multiple nodules on the surface, deep fixation, and clear boundaries. It is a recurrence of abdominal tumor after surgery. The family does not want to undergo surgery and also refuses radiotherapy and chemotherapy.

The patient was to continue to take XZ-C immune-regulating Chinese medicine XZ-C1+4, LMS, MDZ, topical XZ-C3 anti-cancer swelling ointment, and insist on taking the medicine daily until the physical examination at the return visit on February 24, 2002:

The supraclavicular is not buckled and abnormal, the abdomen is soft, can be buckled and the fist is large, hard in quality, deep fixed, with clear edges, but smaller than before, and the condition is stable.

As of December 15, 2004, the re-examination for physical examination was generally good, and the mental appetite was good, but the abdomen was bulging, ascites symptoms, large lumps in the abdomen and adult punches, uneven surface, multiple nodules, deep fixation, no distant position was found Signs of transfer.

After the addition of Xiaoshui Decoction, the ascites subsided. The patient has been taking XZ-C immunomodulatory Chinese medicine for a long time for 5 years. It has been 6 years for the recurrence of abdominal tumor after surgery. The condition is stable, the control has not progressed and increased, and no distant metastasis has occurred. See Figure as the above.

Analysis and Evaluation

This case has a huge liquid tumor in the abdominal cavity, which recurred after resection, and a huge abdominal mass. After 1 cycle of postoperative chemotherapy, the response was large and it was not repeated. In June 1999, he came to the specialist outpatient clinic XZ-C1+3+4 for treatment, long-term oral administration and external application of XZ- C. Immune regulation Chinese medicine has been more than 3 years, and it has been 6 years so far. The condition has been stabilized, no distant metastasis has occurred, the tumor has not increased further, and the tumor has survived.

4. **Extensive bone metastasis, typical cases of more than 3 years treated with XZ-C immunomodulation anti-cancer Chinese medicine**

Case 1

Pan XX, female, 68 years old, from Shenyang

Diagnosis

Multiple bone metastases all over the body after radical mastectomy.

The figure of diagnosis and treatment of bone metastases after breast cancer surgery is as the following:

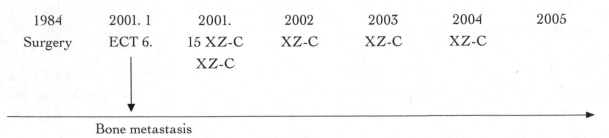

Medical history and treatment

In 1984, patients with right breast cancer underwent radical mastectomy. Pathological diagnosis:

Pure breast cancer, no lymph node metastasis, instigator + MTX chemotherapy for 2 years after surgery, and then every year some drugs to improve the body's immunity.

Consciously felt right shoulder pain in January 2001, ECT found multiple bone metastasis, right supraclavicular lymph node swelling, and 25 radiotherapy was performed on the right supraclavicular lymph node area from March 27. During the radiotherapy, the whole blood cell decreased and the WBC dropped to 2.9 X109/L, symptoms relieved after radiotherapy.

In 2001, the patient took XZ-C immunomodulatory Chinese medicine XZ-C1+4+2, LMS, MDZ on June 15, 2001. After 2 months of long-term medication, the patient's symptoms improved significantly. After taking the medicine for half a year, the ECT returned to normal and my condition was stable.

The patient called on September 2, 2002 and said that the physical examination was normal, especially the ECT examination returned to normal. The patient insisted on taking the medicine every month. I took the XZ-C1 mixture XZ-C4 capsules and XZ-C2 capsules for a long time. It has been 4 years so far. Intermittent.

A phone call from Shenyang in April 2005 said that the patient is generally in good condition, with good mental appetite, and walking activities such as healthy elderly people. The whole body review, liver and gallbladder ultrasound, chest X-ray, ECT showed no abnormalities, and the condition has recovered. See Figure as the above.

Analysis and Evaluation

This patient had a recurrence 17 years after radical mastectomy for right breast cancer, with extensive bone metastases throughout the body, bone destruction and pain in the right shoulder, and improved after radiotherapy. Long-term use of XZ-C immunoregulatory anti-cancer medicine XZ-C1+4+2 which protects Thymus and increase immune function, protects the marrow and produces blood, improves the immune function, and controls extensive bone metastasis throughout the body.

Case 2

Zhong xx, male, 66 years old, from Wuxi, cadre
Medical record number xxxxx

Diagnosis

Right kidney clear cell carcinoma, whole body bone metastasis, supraclavicular metastasis

The figure of diagnosis and treatment of bone metastases from renal cancer is as the following:

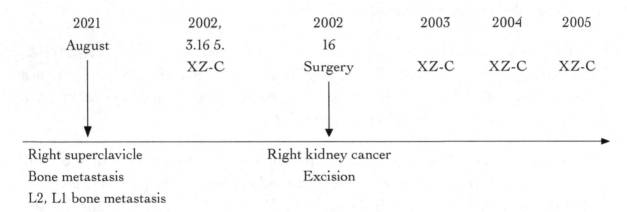

2021	2002,	2002	2003	2004	2005
August	3.16 5.	16			
	XZ-C	Surgery	XZ-C	XZ-C	XZ-C

Right superclavicle   Right kidney cancer
Bone metastasis   Excision
L2, L1 bone metastasis

Medical history and treatment

In August 2001, due to pain in the right shoulder, he was considered to be "frozen shoulder" after examination.

Later, a large walnut mass appeared on the right clavicle near the sternum, and the puncture showed adenocarcinoma cells.

No primary lesions were found by B-ultrasound, CT of the abdomen, chest, and XZ-C immunomodulation and integrated traditional Chinese and Western medicine treatment at the Shuguang Oncology Clinic on March 16, 2002. XZ-C1+4 was taken orally, and XZ- After C3 application, the clavicle mass became softer and slightly shrunk.

On March 24, 2002, B-ultrasound found a 3.1cmX4.2cm CT, L2, L4 parenchymal mass in the right kidney area with bone destruction, using XZ-C 1+4+6 and Gemcitabine (GEM) + cisplatin 1 course of chemotherapy.

Right nephrectomy was performed on May 16, 2002. The tumor of the right kidney was about the size of a table tennis ball. The pathological report was clear cell carcinoma. Due to the large response to chemotherapy, no chemotherapy was performed after the operation. I only took Z-C1+4+2 immunomodulatory drugs. According to the anti-metastasis treatment mode, take XZ-C immunomodulatory anti-cancer drugs daily for a long period of time. After taking the drug, the general condition is good, the spirit and appetite are good, although the whole body has bone metastasis, the walking activities are still normal, 2002, 2003, July 2004, both He came to the clinic every month for follow-up visits and medicines, and his appetite and condition were basically stable.

Until July 2004, suddenly dizzy, easy to forget to speak, and contradictory, CT examination was cerebral hemorrhage, staying in neurology, lying in bed for 3 weeks, CT re-detected blood has been absorbed, continue to take XZ-C1+4+2, LMS, Brucea javanica Treatments such as milk, agrimony granules, solanum granules, Huangmao granules, Huangfen granules, etc., the general condition gradually improved, and the mental appetite improved. See Figure as the above.

Analysis and Evaluation

In August 2001, this patient was found to have metastatic tumors of the right clavicle and L2 and L4 bones. The supraclavicular mass was punctured and found to be metastatic adenocarcinoma. After a comprehensive examination, he was found to be a tumor of the right kidney. On May 16, 2002, he had a right kidney resection. For clear cell carcinoma, XZ-C immunomodulatory anti-cancer medicine was started on March 16, 2002. It was taken orally and externally. The condition was stable for more than 3 years, and no further metastasis was controlled. After taking the medicine, the patient had good appetite and stable condition.

5. **Typical cases that have only been treated with XZ-C anticancer Chinese medicine for 5-11 years, after radical surgery, the patient cannot have radiotherapy and chemotherapy**

Case 1

Ding xx, male, 63 years old, from Wuhan, cadre
Medical record number xxxxx

Diagnosis

Middle Esophageal Cancer

The figure of Diagnosis and treatment of middle esophageal cancer is as the following:

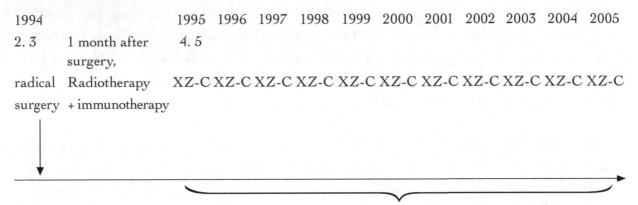

1994		1995 1996 1997 1998 1999 2000 2001 2002 2003 2004 2005
2. 3	1 month after surgery,	4. 5
radical surgery	Radiotherapy + immunotherapy	XZ-C XZ-C XZ-C XZ-C XZ-C XZ-C XZ-C XZ-C XZ-C XZ-C XZ-C

XZ-C1+4 alone, no chemotherapy, 11 years, good health

Medical history and treatment

Progressive dysphagia occurred in January 1994 and was diagnosed by barium swallow examination. On February 3 of the same year, he underwent radical resection of middle esophageal cancer, neck esophagogastric anastomosis, and postoperative radiotherapy for 1 month. Due to heart problems, no postoperative failure With chemotherapy,

On April 5, 1995, he came to the outpatient clinic of the Integrated Chinese and Western Medicine Anti-cancer Cooperation Group, and was treated with XZ-C1+4 immunomodulatory Chinese medicine. After taking the medicine, he had good appetite and physical strength. From 1996 to 1999, he came to the outpatient clinic once a month. Take the medicine, and insist on taking XZ-C1+4 for a long time, in good condition,

At the follow-up visit in July 2005, the patient's hair was gray. In the past year or so, his hair has gradually become black. Now he has black hair, and his facial skin is softer than before. His complexion is rosy. He is a completely healthy old man. It has been 11 years. The patient still taking XZ-C Chinese medicine, Figure as the above.

Analysis and Evaluation

This patient underwent radical mastectomy for middle esophageal cancer on February 3, 1994, and received radiotherapy and immunotherapy 40 days after the operation

After that, he took XZ-C immunoregulatory Chinese medicine for a long time. It has been 11 years and he is in good health.

The treatment experience of this patient is:

Radiotherapy and immunotherapy were done within 40 days after operation.

After 40 days, he will take XZ-C1+4 immune-regulating Chinese medicine for a long time to protect the breast and promote blood.

XZ-C1 can inhibit cancerous cells, and XZ-C4 can promote immunity, induce cancer suppressor factors, improve the overall immune system function, protect immune organs, and eliminate the recurrence factors of dormant cells entering the proliferation stage. Long-term continuous medication keeps the body at a high level of immune function for a long time, prevents recurrence and metastasis, and restores health.

Case 2

Yan xx, female, 71 years old, from Wuhan, teacher
Medical record number xxxxx

Diagnosis

Ascending colon cancer

The figure of ascending colon cancer diagnosis and treatment process is as the following:

1994	1995. 7. 4	1996. 6	1997	1998	1999	2000	2001	2002	2003
12. 19	XZ-C1+4	XZ-C	XZ-C	XZ-C	XZ-C	XZ-C	XZ-C	XZ-C	XZ-C
Surgical resection									

↓

Left low
Lung lobe
Removement

Medical history and treatment

Due to abdominal pain and bloody stools, colon cancer was found under fiber colonoscopy (confirmed by biopsy).

Underwent a radical resection of the right hemicolon on December 19, 1994,

Pathology: Differentiated adenocarcinoma of the colon invades serous membrane. No other treatment was done after the operation.

The patient came to the clinic on July 4, 1995.

The patient adopted XZ-C1+4 immuno-regulatory anti-cancer traditional Chinese medicine as a postoperative adjuvant treatment to prevent postoperative metastasis and recurrence.

After taking XZ-C immune traditional Chinese medicine for a long time, it has been 10 years after the operation, and he is in good health.

Follow-up in April 2005, the old man is 81 years old this year. He is a healthy old man. He still plays cards in the afternoon. See Figure as the above.

Analysis and Evaluation

In this case, after resection of ascending colon cancer, he simply took XZ-C immunoregulatory Chinese medicine as an adjuvant treatment after surgery.

It has been 10 years since the operation, and the condition is good.

This example suggests:

After surgery, supplemented with XZ-C immunoregulatory Chinese medicine treatment, it can strengthen the body to eliminate evil, which can effectively prevent recurrence and metastasis.

Case 3

Zhou xx, male, 49 years old, from Wuhan, cadre
Medical record number xxxxx

Diagnosis

Right lower lobe lung cancer

The figure of the diagnosis and treatment of lung cancer in the lower right lobe was as the following:

1997 4. 28	1997 5. 15	1998	1999	2000	2001	2002	2004. 4
Surgery	XZ-C	XZ-C	XZ-C	XZ-C	XZ-C	XZ-C	XZ-C

Right
lower lobe
Excision

Medical history and treatment

In October 1996, chest tightness, cough, low-grade fever, and dyspnea were treated as "cold" treatment.

He had a sudden hemoptysis in mid-April 1997, and was diagnosed as right lower lobe lung cancer by X-ray chest radiograph and CT examination. On April 28, 1997, he underwent right lower lobe lung resection at Union Hospital.

Pathology: poorly differentiated adenocarcinoma of the lung, with good recovery after operation. No radiotherapy or chemotherapy was done after surgery.

On May 15, 1997, the patient came to the Shuguang Oncology Specialty Clinic to take XZ-C Immunomodulation **Anticancer No. 1, No. 4, No. 7, vitamin C, vitamin B6, vitamin E, and vitamin A.**

After taking the medicine, the general condition is good, the spirit is good, the appetite is good, the complexion is ruddy, and there is no discomfort. After taking the medicine for 3 and a half years, the condition is good, and the condition is stable and controlled without recurrence or metastasis.

On April 6, 2004, the patient came to the clinic and reported that after taking the Z-C immunomodulatory anticancer drug for 3 and a half years, it has been 8 years, and the general condition is very good, just like a healthy person. See Figure as the above.

Analysis and Evaluation

This case is a poorly differentiated adenocarcinoma of the right lower lobe. After surgical resection, no radiotherapy or chemotherapy was performed. After the operation, he came to the outpatient department of Shuguang Oncology Specialty of the Integrated Traditional Chinese and Western Medicine Anticancer Cooperation Group. After taking XZ-C1+4+7, the patient's condition recovered well. Now 8 years after the operation, he has good appetite and good health.

Case 4

Zhang x, male, 52 years old from Wuhan, driver
Medical record number xxxxx

Diagnosis

Right lung poorly differentiated adenocarcinoma, lymph node metastasis

The figure of diagnosis and treatment of poorly differentiated adenocarcinoma of the right lung is as the following:

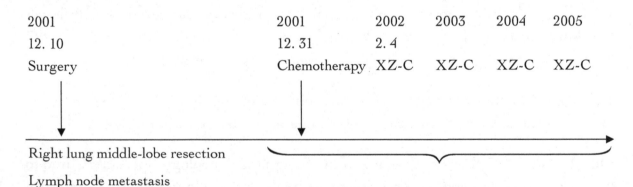

Medical history and treatment

Due to cough and hemoptysis, CT examination showed a tumor of the right lower lung, and there was no abnormality in bronchoscopy.

On December 1, 2001, a thoracotomy was performed at the Provincial Tumor Hospital for resection of the right middle and lower lobes. During the operation, 1 lymph node in the interlobular group and 2 lymph nodes in the hilar group were seen.

The pathological section of the lung is poorly differentiated adenocarcinoma, and the lymph nodes are metastatic adenocarcinoma.

Chemotherapy was performed once after surgery. On February 4, 2002, I came to Shuguang Oncology Specialty Clinic to take XZ-C immunoregulatory anti-cancer and anti-metastasis Chinese medicine treatment.

After taking the medicine, the general condition is good, the mental appetite is good, and the patient had been taking XZ-C1+4+7, LMS, and MDZ daily for a long time for 3 years. The health condition is restored to good condition shown in Figure as the above.

Analysis and Evaluation

This case is a poorly differentiated adenocarcinoma of the right lower lobe with hilar lymph node metastasis. Postoperative chemotherapy was performed once, that is, XZ-C immunomodulator XZ-C1 + XZ-C4 + XZ-C7 was used as postoperative adjuvant treatment.

XZ-C1 kills cancer cells but not normal cells. XZ-C4 protects the thymus, improves immunity, protects the marrow and produces blood, and XZ-C7 protects lung function. Patients have taken XZ-C immunomodulatory drugs for more than 3 years to improve overall immune function. The metastasis was controlled, and no distant metastasis was found. So far, it has been 4 years. The patient is in good condition, has a good appetite, and walks as normal.

Case 5

Yin xx, female, 60 years old Huang Poren
Medical record number xxxxx

Diagnosis

Sigmoid colon cancer, after left hemicolectomy

The figure of treatment after left colectomy for sigmoid colon cancer was as the following:

1999 12,3	2000. 1. 12	2001	2002	2003	2004	2005
Surgery	XZ-C	XZ-C	XZ-C	XZ-C	XZ-C	XZ-C

Z-C1+4, LMS

Medical history and treatment

In August 1998, the stool was bloody, and the local treatment was based on "hemorrhoids".

A colonoscopy was performed at Xiehe Hospital in October 1999, and there was a circular stenosis at 32cm.

On December 3, 1999, the left hemicolon was resected in Union Hospital.

The pathology is as the following:

Papillary tubular adenocarcinoma of the sigmoid colon, which invades the entire intestinal wall, and metastases to mesenteric lymph nodes (6/8),

The patient came to Shuguang Clinic on January 12, 2000 to take XZ-C immune-regulated anti-cancer medicine, Z-C1+4, LMS, MDZ, VT to prevent recurrence and metastasis, and take XZ-C immune-regulated anti-cancer medicine 3 8 months in a year,

On August 4, 2003, his son came to fetch medicine. He said that he was in good condition, doing housework every day, and was in a good mood. He brought more than 10 buckets of water every day to water the flowers, planted various flowers in a large yard, and planted some vegetables. The spirit and appetite are very good.

The patient has always been in a good mood, optimistic mood, and good labor. Always adhere to the Z-C immune regulation Chinese medicine, take the medicine on time and in the amount every day.

This patient did not receive adjuvant chemotherapy after the operation, but only took XZ-C immunotherapy, which was an adjuvant therapy after the operation.

The patient continued to take XZ-C for another 4 months, which has been 5 and a half years. See the Figure as the above.

Analysis and Evaluation

This patient has sigmoid colon cancer and mesenteric lymph node metastasis. After radical surgery, WBC decreased and could not be adjuvant chemotherapy. He was treated with XZ-C immunoregulatory anti-cancer traditional Chinese medicine for postoperative adjuvant treatment, **which was to protect Thymus and increase immune function and to protect bone marrow and to produce the blood, to improve the body's anti-cancer immunity and to** prevent metastasis and recurrence. It has been five and a half years so far, and the situation is generally good.

Case 6

Yu xx, female, 63 years old, from Jilin, cadre
Medical record number xxxxx

Diagnosis

Rectal adenocarcinoma

The figure of diagnosis and treatment of rectal adenocarcinoma was as the following:

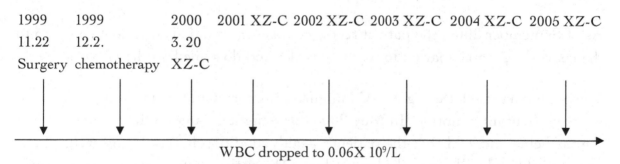

1999	1999		2000	2001 XZ-C	2002 XZ-C	2003 XZ-C	2004 XZ-C	2005 XZ-C
11.22	12.2.		3. 20					
Surgery	chemotherapy		XZ-C					

WBC dropped to 0.06X 10⁹/L

Medical history and treatment

In October 1999, he had blood in the stool, and a large cauliflower-like mass on the fingertips 10 cm away from the anus was examined by a rectal microscope. The pathological biopsy section showed rectal adenocarcinoma.

On November 22, 1999, he underwent a radical resection of rectal cancer in the affiliated hospital with Dixon operation and recovered well.

On December 2, intraperitoneal chemotherapy (5-FU1.0, 1 time/d, for 5 days, carboplatin 100mg once/d, for 3 days), WBC dropped to 0. 09X10^9/L on December 9.

On December 10, WBC dropped to 0.06X10^9/L, 5 days after injection of white blood cell-boosting medicine, WBC rose to 1. 1X10^9/L, lung infection, persistent high fever up to 40^{0}C.

On January 2, 2000, I used Tynene + ciprofloxacin, but the fever still persists, and my throat is infected with 3 kinds of bacteria. The patient can't eat or drink water.

After using "Dafukang" for 5 days, the body temperature dropped to 38^{0}C, and the patient had pulmonary heart disease, high blood pressure and mild diabetes. At this point, the patient was extremely weak and in critical condition. He was critically ill twice.

He improved after 2 months of treatment. On March 20, 2000, the patient came to the anti-cancer clinic of Integrative Chinese and Western Medicine, treated with XZ-C immunomodulatory Chinese medicine. After 2 months of taking XZ-C1+4+LMS, the patient's appetite and general condition improved, could get up and half a year after taking XZ-C medicine, the general condition has improved significantly, and he could take care of himself and do some housework.

As of September 2000, the patient recovery was very good. The patient could go to the nearby vegetable market to buy vegetables and do some light housework.

The patient has been taking XZ-C immunoregulatory Chinese medicine daily for 5 years without interruption. In May 2005, his daughter came to the clinic to collect the medicine and said that the patient's health condition is recovering well. She is 68 years old and still doing the house chore. The patient still does some housework, just like other healthy elderly people. See Figure as the above.

Analysis and Evaluation

After radical resection of rectal cancer and intraperitoneal chemotherapy, this patient's immune function and bone marrow hematopoietic function were severely inhibited. This caused serious infection of the throat and both lungs, followed by a double fungal infection.

After treatment, the patient continued to take immuno-regulating Chinese medicine for a longer period of time.

XZ-Cl only inhibits cancer cells, does not affect normal cells, and strengthens the body.

XZ- C4 protects Thymus and promotes immunity, and protects bone marrow and promotes the recovery of overall immune function.

Chemotherapy cytotoxic drugs inhibit bone marrow, which actually leads to varying degrees of bone marrow aplasia. The effect can sometimes last as long as 2-3 years.

Therefore, the XZ-C immunomodulatory drug that protects the Thymus and protects the marrow and produces blood needs to be taken for several years in order to facilitate the complete recovery of immune function and bone marrow hematopoietic function.

Case 7

Peng xxxxx, female, 39 years old, from Leshan, Sichuan, cadre
Medical record number xxxxx

Diagnosis

Thyroid cancer

The figure of diagnosis and treatment of thyroid cancer was as the following:

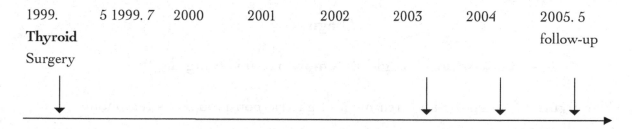

1999.	5 1999. 7	2000	2001	2002	2003	2004	2005. 5
Thyroid							follow-up
Surgery							

Medical history and treatment

The right neck mass was removed on April 27, 1999, and the postoperative examination was (thyroid) follicular papillary carcinoma with focal lymphocytic thyroiditis.

Radical thyroid cancer surgery was performed on May 6, 1999. After the operation, the voice was hoarse, but radiotherapy and chemotherapy were not performed.

Came to Shuguang Oncology Clinic on July 24, 1999 to take XZ-C immunomodulatory Chinese medicine XZ-C1 +XZ-C4, LMS, VS postoperative adjuvant treatment, monthly follow-up visits, continuous XZ-C immunomodulatory drugs for half a year.

By January 2000, the voice gradually improved, and after another 3 months of taking XZ-C, the voice gradually returned to normal.

The general condition is good, the mental appetite is good, the physical strength is restored, and he resumes work. He insists on taking XZ-C1+4 for a long time to improve the overall immune function. It has been 6 years so far, and he went back to the clinic in May 2005 and is in good health. See Figure as the above.

Analysis and Evaluation

This case is thyroid follicular papillary carcinoma. The patient has severe hoarseness occurred after radical operation. The patient didn't have postoperative adjuvant treatment such as radiotherapy or chemotherapy was performed. XZ-C immunoregulatory Chinese medicine was simply taken orally to improve overall immunity function to prevent recurrence and metastasis by the patient.

Case 8

Liu xx, female, 34 years old, from NSW
Medical record number xxxxxx

Diagnosis

Gastric non-Hodgkin's lymphoma, involving the liver

The figure of diagnosis and treatment of gastric non-Hodgkin's lymphoma was as the following:

1999	1999	2000	2001	2002	2003	2004	2005
6.29 8. Surgery	18 XZ-C	XZ-C	XZ-C	XZ-C	XZ-C	XZ-C	

XZ-C Chinese Medicine

Medical history and treatment

There was a sense of obstruction after eating in February 1999, which was not taken seriously.

By April, the symptoms of obstruction were more obvious, and drinking and liquid food were also obstructed.

Gastroscopy in May showed cancer of the gastric body and Guimen,

A total gastrectomy was performed at Xiehe Hospital on June 29.

The pathological section is: non-Hodgkin's lymphoma of the stomach, involving liver tissue, spleen and stomach large and small curved lymph nodes.

Because of her weakness, she did not receive chemotherapy or other treatments after surgery,

On August 18, 1999, he came to Shuguang Oncology Specialty Clinic to take XZ-C immunoregulatory anti-cancer Chinese medicine XZ-C1+4 as a postoperative adjuvant treatment.

After taking the medicine for 2 months, the general condition is good, the spirit and appetite are good. He has been taking XZ-C medicine daily for 3 years, and the abdominal B-ultrasound is reviewed every year, and there is no abnormality.

After November 2002, she felt that she was in good condition, with good mental appetite and physical strength, so she changed to taking XZ-C medicine intermittently.

On January 18, 2004, when he came to the clinic for follow-up visit, he was generally in good condition, had good mental appetite, flat, soft, unbuckled and abnormal abdomen. However, the left hand was sometimes weak, but the left hand was active and the grip was normal, and he could do housework.

The follow-up visit in April 2005, the general condition was good, no discomfort, and it is required to take XZ-C1+4 intermittently for a long time to consolidate the long-term effect. See Figure as the above.

Analysis and Evaluation

This case is gastric non-Hodgkin's lymphoma, involving liver tissue, spleen, stomach large and small curved lymph nodes. After total gastrectomy, because the body is thin and weak, the patient doesn't have chemotherapy after surgery, the patient only has XZ-C$_{1+4}$ immune regulation and control adjuvant therapy, strengthening the body and improving immunity, improve the overall immune function, and promote the recovery of patients after surgery. After the operation, the patients adhere to the long-term daily oral XZ-C immunomodulatory adjuvant therapy to prevent recurrence and metastasis, thereby consolidating the long-term effect. It has been nearly 6 years.

Case 9

He x, male, 76 years old, from Henan, cadre
Medical record number xxxxxx

Diagnosis

Left kidney lower pole clear cell carcinoma

The figure of diagnosis and treatment of left renal clear cell carcinoma is as the following:

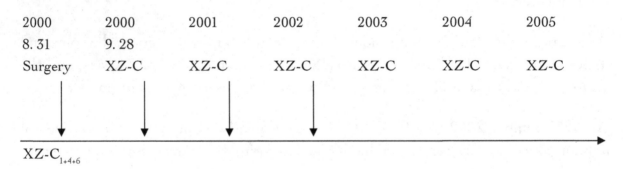

2000	2000	2001	2002	2003	2004	2005
8. 31	9. 28					
Surgery	XZ-C	XZ-C	XZ-C	XZ-C	XZ-C	XZ-C

XZ-C$_{1+4+6}$

Medical history and treatment

In 1996, there was a kidney cyst. In 2000, the left kidney cyst was 7.5cmX6.5cm on physical examination. CT and MRI were performed for left kidney tumor. The left nephrectomy was performed at Tongji Hospital on August 31, 2000.

Pathology report:

Moderately differentiated clear cell renal cell carcinoma, after taking medroxyprogesterone acetate, without radiotherapy or chemotherapy,

He came to Shuguang Oncology Clinic on September 28, 2000, and used XZ-C1+4+6 immune-regulated anti-cancer Chinese medicine to protect breasts and promote blood circulation.

After taking the medicine for 1 month, the spirit is good, the sleep is good, and the appetite is poor. After taking the medicine for 3 months, the general condition is good, the spirit and appetite are good, and the sleep is good.

After taking the medicine for a reexamination one year later, the abdominal B-ultrasound, chest X-ray and various routine laboratory tests were all normal. Continue to take XZ-C1+4+6 immunoregulatory Chinese medicine to prevent recurrence and metastasis.

It has been 5 years so far, and the health condition has recovered well. The follow-up visit on April 10, 2005, is generally in good condition, with red light on the face, loud voice, good energy, slightly fat, and presbycusis. The health status should be 100 points according to the Carrok score., Re-examination of CT, chest X-ray, liver and gallbladder ultrasound, liver and kidney function, and blood biochemistry are all normal, but the prostatic hypertrophy is shown in Figure as the above.

Analysis and Evaluation

This case was a clear cell carcinoma of the left kidney. He was 76 years old at the time of surgery. Due to his frail age, he did not undergo radiotherapy or chemotherapy after the operation, and only used XZ-C immunoregulatory Chinese medicine as an adjuvant treatment after the operation to protect Thymus and to promote immunity, to protect the bone marrow and to produce the blood, and to improve overall immune function to prevent recurrence and metastasis.

The patient has been taking XZ-C immunomodulatory drugs for a long time for 5 years. The patient is 80 years old this year. The patient is in good general condition, good appetite, red face and full of energy. The voice is loud, for a healthy old man.

Case 10

Chen xx, female, 44 years old, from Wuhan
Medical record number xxxxxx

Diagnosis

Breast cancer

The figure of the process of breast cancer diagnosis and treatment is as the following:

1995		1995. 5. 11	1996	1997	1998	1999	2000	2001	2002
2. 20		Postoperative	XZ-C	XZ-C	XZ-C	XZ-C	XZ-C	XZ-C	XZ-C	XZ-C
Right breast		radiotherapy							
cancer surgery		1 course of radical							
		operation							
		is not finished							

Take XZ-C continuously   Intermittent taking

Medical history and treatment

Found a right breast mass for 3 months, puncture confirmed breast cancer,

Radical mastectomy was performed on February 20, 1995.

1 course of postoperative radiotherapy, due to poor physical strength, could not continue,

He came to the collaborative group clinic on May 11, 1995 and was treated with XZ-C1+4.

After taking XZ-C Chinese medicine for a long time for nearly 3 years, the patient has good appetite, weight gain, physical recovery, and outpatient checkup once a month. After that, he takes XZ-C immunoregulatory Chinese medicine intermittently every year. The whole body is in good condition. Other treatments. See Figure as the above.

Analysis and Evaluation

This patient underwent radical mastectomy on February 20, 1995, and received 1 course of postoperative radiotherapy. Due to poor physical strength, he could not continue.

It came to the collaborative group clinic on May 11, 1995 to use XZ-C and immune regulation Chinese medicine as an adjuvant treatment after surgery. After taking the medicine for more than 3 years, and then taking XZ-C medicine intermittently, the patient is in good condition, without chemotherapy, and has been in good health for nearly 10 years.

Case 11

Li xx, female, 33 years old, from Changde, Hunan, worker
Medical record number xxxxxx

Diagnosis

Simple left breast cancer

The figure of process of diagnosis and treatment of simple breast cancer is as the following:

1996	1996	1996	1997	1997	1998	1999	2001	2002	2003
11.29	12. 25	12. 29	04.02	5. 14	XZ-C	XZ-C	XZ-C	XZ-C	XZ-C
Radical surgery	XZ-C chemotherapy	CMF	radiotherapy	radiotherapy 25 times					

XZ-C1+4 + no response to radiotherapy and chemotherapy

After June 1997, the patient did not undergo radiotherapy and chemotherapy. It has been 6 and a half years since only using XZ-C drugs. He is in good health. He comes to Wuchang from Changde for follow-up visits every 3 months, His life is like the normal people

Medical history and treatment

Radical mastectomy for breast cancer was performed in Changde on November 29, 1996, and the right axillary lymph node metastasis ((3/5), CMF regimen chemotherapy was given one month after the operation, once a week for 4 weeks.

On December 25, 1996, the collaborative group was treated with XZ-C series of drugs to protect the marrow and produce blood. After taking the medicine, the appetite is good and the blood picture rises.

From April 2, 1997 to May 14, 1997, 4 months after right breast cancer surgery + 15 times of radiotherapy on the inner side of the right breast, 15 times on the right axillary, and 25 times on the outer side of the right breast. During the radiotherapy, z-C was used in conjunction with treatment, and there was no response.

After taking the XZ-C drug, the patient has been better after radiotherapy and chemotherapy, and the response is very mild, and there is basically no response.

After June 2004, the patient did not undergo radiotherapy or chemotherapy. The patient has been taking XZ-C series of medicines. The patient returns this clinic from Changde every 3 months and refills XZ-C medicines for 3 months. He persists for a long time and has good results.

He came for follow-up visit in December 2004. The general condition is good, the appetite is good, the complexion is ruddy, the activities are as normal, and he can do housework. The patient travels from Changde to Wuchang every three months, as if he is healthy. See Figure as the above.

Analysis and Evaluation

The treatment experience of this patient:

1. Using XZ-C4 during radiotherapy and chemotherapy can reduce the response, and it can be used to consolidate the long-term effect and prevent recurrence during the intermittent period of radiotherapy and chemotherapy.

2. Six months after the operation, radiotherapy and chemotherapy + XZ-C Chinese medicine not only attack the residual cancer cells or residual small cancer foci, but also protect the host and immune organs.

After half a year, the general condition is good, that is, use the XZ-C series to strengthen the body to eliminate evil and consolidate the long-term efficacy. It has been 9 years since the operation, XZ-Cimmune regulation and control Chinese medicine can consolidate the long-term effect.

Case 12

Liu xx, female, 49 years old, from Wuhan, accountant
Medical record number xxxxxx

Diagnosis

Left breast ductal carcinoma

The figure of the diagnosis and treatment of breast ductal carcinoma is as the following:

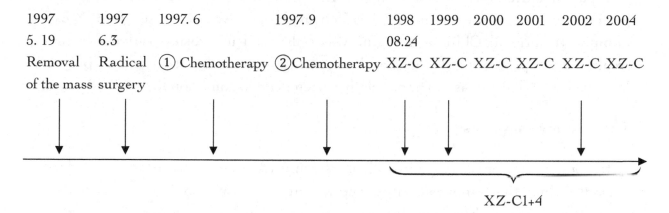

1997	1997	1997. 6	1997. 9	1998	1999	2000	2001	2002	2004
5. 19	6.3			08.24					
Removal of the mass	Radical surgery	① Chemotherapy	②Chemotherapy	XZ-C	XZ-C	XZ-C	XZ-C	XZ-C	XZ-C

XZ-C1+4

Medical history and treatment

On May 19, 1997, because the left breast mass was 3cmX 3cm, the left breast mass was removed, and the section was left breast invasive ductal carcinoma.

The operation was performed again on June 3, 1997, and radical mastectomy was performed for left breast cancer. No residual cancer was found in the residual breast tissue, and no metastasis was found in the ipsilateral axillary lymph nodes. Chemotherapy was used twice after the operation. The oral Miflon reaction was severe and did not continue.

On August 24, 1997, he came to the outpatient clinic of the Anti-Cancer Cooperation Group of Integrated Traditional Chinese and Western Medicine, and was supplemented with XZ-C immunoregulatory Chinese medicine treatment after the operation. After taking the medicine, he was generally in good condition and had a good appetite.

After 3 months, he returned to health as a normal person and resumed work,

Four months later, two masses of 3cmx3cm in size were found in the right breast, with unclear borders. Puncture cytology showed breast hyperplasia.

The patient used XZ-C1+4+ Mammary Gland Hyperplasia and Elimination Decoction. In the past 3 years, the patient only used XZ-C immunize Chinese medicine. The condition is good and the work is as usual. See Figure as the above.

Analysis and Evaluation

This patient suffered from breast cancer. After radical operation, chemotherapy was performed twice. Since August 24, 1997, chemotherapy was no longer used. XZ-C immune traditional Chinese medicine was only used for postoperative adjuvant treatment for protecting Thymus and increasing immune function and to protect Recurrence and metastasis. The patient has been in good condition for nearly 8 years.

This example suggests:

After breast cancer surgery, two chemotherapy treatments are used for a short period of time, the response is large, and it cannot be done anymore. Later, XZ-C immunoregulatory Chinese medicine is used as an adjuvant treatment after surgery.

XZ-C1+4 can induce endogenous anti-cancer factors, induce differentiation, and improve the overall Immune function, protect and improve the host's anti-cancer ability.

Case 13

Qian x, male, 66 years old, from Wuhan, senior accountant
Medical record number xxxxxx

Diagnosis

Rectal adenocarcinoma

The Figure of Diagnosis and treatment of rectal adenocarcinoma is as the following:

1998 1.24 Dixon surgery	1998. 3. 3 XZ-C	1999 XZ-C	1999. 12 XZ-C	2000. 5 XZ-C	2001 XZ-C	2002 XZ-C	2003 XZ-C	2004 XZ-C

XZ-C1+4, LMS

Medical history and treatment

Intermittent diarrhea, constipation for 2 years, stool with blood, anal digital examination of the knee and chest at 6 points was to touch a 3cmX 3cm mass.

On January 20, 1998, fiber colonoscopy showed malignant transformation of rectal polyps.

On January 24, 1998, a Dixon operation was performed at Xiehe Hospital to remove 40 cm of the colon.

The pathological section showed a rectal tubular adenocarcinoma, moderately differentiated, invading the superficial muscle layer of the intestinal wall, no lymph node metastasis was found, and no cancer was found at the cut end.

After no chemotherapy, he came to the clinic on March 3, 1998. He was treated with XZ-C immunomodulatory Chinese medicine alone. He took XZ-C medicine for a long time for nearly 8 years. He has been back to work for 5 years without discomfort.

Continue to take XZ-C immune regulation Chinese medicine. See Figure as the above.

Analysis and Evaluation

This patient was a rectal adenocarcinoma. The pathological section of the patient underwent Dixon radical resection in January 1998 to be a rectal tubular adenocarcinoma, moderately differentiated, no chemotherapy after surgery, and XZ-C1+4 immunoregulatory Chinese medicine alone as a postoperative adjuvant The treatment has been in good condition for the past 8 years.

This example suggests

Radical treatment of rectal cancer after Dixon surgery, without chemotherapy, XZ-C immunomodulation Chinese medicine alone, breast protection and immunization, and marrow protection, improve postoperative immunity, enhance the patient's disease resistance, and improve the quality of life and prevented recurrence and metastasis, and the condition is good.

Case 14

Yang xx, female, 32 years old, from Zaoyang, accountant
Medical record number xxxxx

Diagnosis

Rectal villous tubular adenocarcinoma

The figure of diagnosis and treatment process of rectal villous tubular adenocarcinoma
is as the following:

1997	1997. 12	1999	2000	2001	2002	2003	2004
9. 17	XZ-C	XZ-C	XZ-C	XZ-C	XZ-C	XZ-C	XZ-C
Surgery							

XZ-C1+4

Medical history and treatment

The stool was bloody, and the biopsy of the rectal microscope in September 1997
was rectal cancer.

Underwent a radical resection of rectal cancer on September 17, 1997,

The tumor is 4cm from the anus, the base is about 1.0cmX1.0cm in size,

The postoperative pathology report was a rectal villous tubular adenocarcinoma,
which invaded the entire thickness of the tube wall and metastasized to mesenteric
lymph nodes.

Chemotherapy was performed once after surgery, but no more chemotherapy was
done because of the significant decrease in white blood cells.

On December 3, 1997, he came to the outpatient clinic of the Anti-cancer Collaborative
Group of Integrated Traditional Chinese and Western Medicine and used XZ-C
immunoregulatory Chinese medicine for treatment.

After taking XZ-C1+4, the general condition is good, the mental appetite is good, and the blood condition is restored. It has been nearly 8 years since XZ-C Chinese medicine has been taken for a long time. He has not undergone other radiotherapy or chemotherapy, and his recovery is good. The housework is like a normal person. See Figure as the above.

Analysis and Evaluation

This patient underwent a radical resection of rectal cancer on September 17, 1997. During the operation, the mesenteric lymph node metastasis was seen, and the cancer invaded the entire thickness of the bowel wall. Chemotherapy was performed once after the operation, and the response was large, and no further treatment was done. From December 3, 1997, the patient came to the Shuguang Oncology Clinic of the Anti-Cancer Cooperation Group of Integrated Traditional Chinese and Western Medicine, and only used XZ-C immune regulation and control anti-cancer Chinese medicine as a postoperative adjuvant treatment to prevent postoperative recurrence and metastasis. It has been 8 years since the long-term medication, and the health recovery is good.

Case 15

Yu XX, male, 69 years old, from Heilongjiang, cadre
Medical record number xxxxx

Diagnosis

Transitional cell carcinoma of the bladder

The figure of diagnosis and treatment of transitional cell carcinoma of the bladder is as the following:

1998.03	1998, 5		1998 XZ-C	1999 XZ-C	2000	2001	2002	XZ-C	2003	2004
Surgery	Once				XZ-C	XZ-C			XZ-C	XZ-C
	Chemotherapy									

XZ-C1+4

Medical history and treatment

Hematuria was found on February 27, 1998,

On March 2nd, cystoscopy and B-ultrasound showed a circular mass on the anterior wall of the bladder, with a size of 1.6cmX1.4cm, protruding into the bladder cavity, which was a new organism on the anterior wall of the bladder.

On March 10, 1998, the tumor tissue in the bladder was removed. The pathological section showed transitional cell carcinoma of the bladder. The doctor told him that the tumor was prone to recurrence.

Chemotherapy was performed once (May 26, 1998) after the operation. The reaction was severe, nausea, vomiting, general malaise, and the left testicle was significantly enlarged. Chemotherapy was stopped.

On June 18, 1998, I came to the Shuguang Oncology Clinic of the Anti-Cancer Cooperation Group of Integrated Traditional Chinese and Western Medicine, treated with XZ-C series of drugs, and came to the outpatient clinic for review every month. The general condition is good, the urine is normal, and no other treatment has been used. For more than a year, no abnormalities were seen. See Figure as the above.

Analysis and Evaluation

This patient was operated on March 10, 1998, and 3 pieces of tumor tissue in the bladder were removed. The pathological section showed transitional cell carcinoma of the bladder. The postoperative chemotherapy was performed once. The reaction was severe. He did not receive chemotherapy again. He came to China on June 18, 1998. In the outpatient clinic of the Anti-Cancer Collaborative Group of Integrated Western Medicine, XZ-C1+4+6 immune traditional Chinese medicine has been used for treatment. It has been in good health for more than 7 years and has not been treated by other methods, and no recurrence or metastasis has been seen.

Case 16

Zhang xx, female, 39 years old, from Wuhan, accounting disease
Calendar number xxxxx

Diagnosis

Carcinogenesis of gastric ulcer, poorly differentiated adenocarcinoma

The figure of diagnosis and treatment of poorly differentiated gastric adenocarcinoma is as the following:

1994. 4. 20		1995. 11. 22	1996	1997	1998	1999	2000	2005
surgery	Postoperative chemotherapy 6 times	XZ-C	XZ-C	XZ-C	XZ-C	XZ-C	XZ-C	XZ-C

XZ-Cl+4+8

Medical history and treatment

In March 1994, due to epigastric discomfort for 1 month and worsening for 1 week, gastroscope showed gastric ulcer.

On April 20, 1994, he underwent a subtotal gastrectomy, 6 postoperative chemotherapy, 5-FU+ MMC liver protection treatment, postoperative pathological section of poorly differentiated gastric cancer, lymph node metastasis.

On November 22, 1995, he came to the outpatient clinic of the Anti-cancer Research Cooperation Group of Integrated Traditional Chinese and Western Medicine to use z-cl+48 immune regulation anti-cancer Chinese medicine. No other treatments were used. Long-term medication was used to promote the immune function and to protect bone marrow. It has been more than 10 years to provent recurrence and metastasis. The patient is in good condition. See Figure as the above.

Analysis and Evaluation

This patient has poorly differentiated adenocarcinoma of the stomach with lymph node metastasis.

He underwent subtotal gastrectomy on April 20, 1994, and received 6 postoperative chemotherapy.

Since November 22, 1995, XZ-C1+4+8 immunomodulatory Chinese medicine has been used only, and no other medicine has been used for treatment. It has been 10 years and the condition is good.

__This example prompts:__

__Postoperative chemotherapy + long-term use of XZ-immune-regulating and controlling cancer suppressor medicine can improve the long-term efficacy.__

__XZ-C immunoregulatory anti-cancer Chinese medicine can prevent postoperative recurrence and metastasis.__

Case 17

Liu XX, 65 years old, from Wuhan, economist
Medical record number: xxxxxx

Diagnosis

Gastric cardia cancer

The figure of diagnosis and treatment of gastric cardia adenocarcinoma is as the following:

1995. 01	1996.03	1997	1998	1999	2000	2001	2002 XZ-C	2003 XZ-C
Surgery	XZ-C	XZ-C	XZ-C	XZ-C	XZ-C	XZ-C		

XZ-C1+4

Medical history and treatment

In January 1995, he was diagnosed with gastric cardia adenocarcinoma by gastroscopy due to stomach pain for half a year in January 1995. Radical gastrectomy was performed, proximal gastrectomy, and esophagogastric anastomosis.

The postoperatively was fine, due to poor physical strength and weight loss, chemotherapy is not suitable.

He came to the Integrative Chinese and Western Medicine Anti-Cancer Collaborative Group on March 16, 1996 for the treatment of biological immunity with traditional Chinese medicine. It was only treated with XZ-C1+4 immunotherapy, and XZ-C was taken continuously for 5 years. Afterwards, the intermittent medication was generally in good condition. Use other treatments. See Figure as the following.

Analysis and Evaluation

This patient had a proximal gastrectomy and gastroesophageal anastomosis in January 1995 for this patient with gastric cardia cancer. He was not suitable for chemotherapy because of his weakness and weight loss. After the operation, he has been treated with XZ-C1+4 immune traditional Chinese medicine for more than 10 years. The general condition is good.

This case suggests that XZ-C immunoregulatory anti-cancer Chinese medicine can prevent recurrence and metastasis after surgery, and the effect is better.

Case 18

Huang xx, male, 66 years old, Huangpi, cadre
Medical record number xxxxx

Diagnosis

Middle and Lower Esophagus Cancer

The figure of diagnosis and treatment of middle and lower esophagus cancer is as the following:

1996. 3	1996. 5	1996.	1997	1998	1999	2000	2001	2002	2003	2004	2005. 4
GI	Surgery	6. 19									
		XZ-C	XZ-C	XZ-C	XZ-C	XZ-C	XZ-C	XZ-C	XZ-C	XZ-C	XZ-C

Continuous monthly medication   Intermit taking medication   In good condition

Medical history and treatment

The patient has the eating obstruction in March 1996, barium meal in late April to diagnose cancer of the middle and lower esophagus.

Radical surgery for esophageal cancer was performed in Union Hospital in May 1996.

No other treatment was done after the operation.

On June 19, 1996, I came to the Specialty Clinic of the Collaboration Group, and used XZ-C immunomodulatory Chinese medicine as a postoperative adjuvant treatment to prevent recurrence and metastasis.

Simply take XZ-C immune-regulating Chinese medicine to protect the thymus gland to promote immunity and the bone marrow to produce blood.

I have been taking XZ-C immune traditional Chinese medicine every day for 3 years, and then I will take it intermittently. After taking the medicine, my general condition is good, my appetite is good, and my walking activities resume as normal.

Follow-up in April 2005, the patient recovered well and often played cards in the afternoon. See Figure as the above.

Analysis and Evaluation

In this case, radiotherapy and chemotherapy were not used after the operation of esophageal cancer, and only Z-c immunoregulatory Chinese medicine was used as an adjuvant treatment after the operation. It has been 9 years and the recovery is good.

The above case tips:

(1) After the operation, XZ-C immune regulation Chinese medicine is supplemented for adjuvant treatment after radical mastectomy. It protects the thymus glands to enhance immunity, protects the marrow to produce blood, protects the central immune organs, improves the patient's overall immune function level, is conducive to patient recovery, and prevents cancer recurrence, Transfer.

(2) The above cases have persisted in taking XZ-C immunomodulatory Chinese medicine for many years. After taking the medicine, they are generally in good condition, have good mental appetite, and have good long-term effects.

It is implying that:

XZ-C immune regulation Chinese medicine is safe and effective, and no obvious side effects have been seen after long-term use.

How to evaluate the efficacy of adjuvant treatment after radical cancer surgery?

It is impossible to use tumor size as an indicator, because the cancer was removed.

Good quality of life and long survival time should be used as indicators.

For the cases exemplified above, XZ-C immunomodulatory adjuvant therapy has been performed for more than 5-11 years, and the recovery is good.

6. **Typical cases of chemotherapy plus XZ-C traditional Chinese medicine in the treatment of acute lymphocytic leukemia**

Case

Zhao xx female 34 years old Wuhan cadre
Medical record number xxxxxx

Diagnosis

Acute lymphocytic leukemia

The figure of diagnosis and treatment of acute lymphocytic leukemia is as the following:

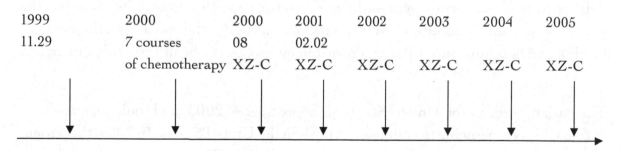

1999	2000	2000	2001	2002	2003	2004	2005
11.29	7 courses of chemotherapy	08 XZ-C	02.02 XZ-C	XZ-C	XZ-C	XZ-C	XZ-C

Acute
Lymphoblastic
leukemia (ALL)

Autologous
peripheral blood stem cell
transplantation

Medical history and treatment

The patient was hospitalized in Beijing People's Hospital on November 1, 1999 due to the diagnosis of "acute lymphoblastic leukemia".

After strengthening and consolidating 7 courses of chemotherapy, autologous peripheral blood stem cell transplantation was performed in August 2000.

However, hematopoietic recovery after transplantation was not ideal, and the three blood lines were low WBC 0.5 X 109 / L, PLT5 X 109 / L, Hb 46g / L.

All rely on fresh blood transfusion, 250 ml of blood transfusion every 8-9 days.

During hospitalization in Beijing, the patient had 10 times of blood transfusion and 14 times of platelet transfusion (an average of 10 days).

He returned to Wuhan from Beijing in February 2001 and came to Shuguang Oncology Clinic for treatment on February 2.

XZ-C1, XZ-C4, XZ-C2, XZ-C8 in XZ-C Immunomodulation Chinese medicines

Have Thymus protection and increase immune function and protect the marrow to produce blood, until April 2001, white blood cells, red blood cells, and platelets gradually increased.

He gradually stopped the transfusion of fresh blood and platelets and was completely treated with XZ-C immunomodulatory Chinese medicine.

Adhere to the long-term 1 year and 7 months, the condition gradually recovers, the general condition is good now, the complexion is ruddy, the spirit appetite is good, talking and laughing and walking like ordinary people, the health condition recovers,

The patient went to the United States on September 4, 2003, and took six months of XZ-C Chinese medicine to continue taking it in the United States. In 2004, the patient emigrated to Canada again, and continued to take XZ-C1+ 4+ 2 immunomodulatory Chinese medicine and Shengxue decoction for a long time. It was sent every 3 months. The patient called from Canada in April 2005. The condition is generally good and spirited Good appetite, good sleep, engaged in commercial work, no physical discomfort, and recovered well. See the figure as the above.

Analysis and evaluation

This patient is acute lymphocytic leukemia. After 7 courses of intensive chemotherapy, autologous peripheral blood stem cell transplantation was performed in August 2000.

The recovery after transplantation was unsatisfactory, the three lines of blood were low, and relied on transfusion of fresh blood and platelets.

On February 2, 2001, he started taking Chinese traditional medicines such as XZ-C1 + XZ-C4 + XZ-C2 and Shengxue Tang.

After taking the medicine for 4 months, the blood gradually picked up,

After 1 year and 7 months, the patient's blood picture and health have improved significantly. So far, he has been taking XZ-C traditional Chinese medicine for 4 years. The patient's health has recovered well, he is engaged in commercial work, and his physical and mental discomfort is satisfactory.

Experience

Chemotherapy for leukemia XZ-C immune regulation Chinese medicine protects the marrow and promotes blood circulation and raises the risk of recovery, which can achieve satisfactory long-term results. The substance of this case may be immunochemotherapy. It has been 7 years so far and it is recovering well.

17

The immune function of Chinese herbal medicine in advanced cancer

1. **Drugs that can improve immune function should be used in the treatment of advanced cancer**

    (1). The findings from tumor experimental research

    Mice with advanced cancer all have low immune function and progressive atrophy of thymus or progressive thymus shrinkage.

    1)). In 1986, when the thymus glands (THC) were removed in the experiment of making tumor-bearing animal models in our laboratory, *the tumor-bearing animal models can be made, and the injection of immunosuppressants can also help the establishment of tumor-bearing animal models.* Or when our laboratory conducted an experiment to create a tumor-bearing animal model, we excised the thymus (TH, Th) to produce a tumor-bearing animal model. Injection of immunosuppressants can also help to establish tumor-bearing animal models.

    The conclusion of the study clearly proves *that the occurrence and development of cancer have a clear positive relationship with the host's immune function and immune organ tissue function*.

    It is difficult to make animal models without removing the thymus.

    Repeatedly repeating the experiment many times, all of these confirmed the experimental results.

2)). After all, is the immune function weakened first and then it is easy to get cancer? Or is it to get cancer first and then it weakens immune function; or whether is the immune function lowering or weak or decreasing first and then the body easy to get cancer, or does the cancer occur first and then the immune function becomes weak or decreasing?

Our experimental results are:

The immune is weak first and then the cancer is easy to occur, if there is no decline in immune function, it is not easy to succeed in vaccination or inolucation.

The results of this study suggest

that improving and maintaining good immune function and protecting the immune organ Thymus (TH) are one of the important measures to prevent cancer.

3)). The Animal models of liver metastasis established in our laboratory to study the relationship between cancer metastasis and immunity are divided into two groups, A and B, with immunosuppressive agents in group A and not in group B.

The Results are the following:

The number of intrahepatic metastases in group A was significantly higher than that in group B.

The suggestion or implication of the results of this experiment are the following:

that metastasis is related to immune function; and that the immunological function is low or the application of immunosuppressive agents may promote tumor metastasis.

4)). When our laboratory conducted experiments to explore the impact of tumors on the immune organs of the body or on the body's immune organs, it was found that as the cancer progresses, TH shows that progressive cell proliferation is blocked and the volume or size is significantly reduced.

The suggestion or implication from these results of this experiment is as the following:

that tumors can inhibit Thymus or TH and cause immune organs to shrink or atrophy.

The above experimental results prove:

a. The occurrence, development, and metastasis of cancer have an obvious positive or certain relationship with the decline of the host's immune function.

b. Late-stage cancers in mice have weakened immune function and progressive Thymu atrophy.

__Therefore, in the treatment of advanced cancer, drugs that increase immune function should be used, but drugs that reduce or suppress immune function should not be used.__

(2). The Experimental Study of searching or looking for medications or drugs that increase immune function and inhibit tumor from the natural medicines and Chinese herbal medicines

*The above experimental results prove that as the tumor progresses, the host's Thymus shows progressive atrophy. So, **can we adopt or use some methods to prevent the host's Thyrnus from atrophy?***

When we were exploring ways to stop the atrophy of the immune organs during tumor progression, to find ways to restore TH to function well, and to rebuild immunity, it was to look for anti-cancer drugs that increase immune function from natural medicines.

200 kinds of traditional Chinese herbal medicines which were traditionally considered to be "anti-cancer traditional Chinese medicines" were screened for tumor-suppressing animals after a long period of time, in batches in our laboratory.

As a result, it was found that 152 species were ineffective, and only 48 species did have a certain or even better inhibitory effect on cancer cell proliferation, as well as an effect of increasing immune function.

Among them, 26 kinds of Chinese herbal medicines (HM) have the function of enhancing macrophages or stimulating the weight increase of the thymus of the animal's immune organs, or increasing white blood cells; or it can promote the proliferation of splenic lymphocytes, increase the rate of lymphocyte transformation, enhance the immune function of T cells, enhance the activity of NK cells, and promote the induction of interferon. After optimizing the combination, through in vivo tumor suppression experiments of tumor-bearing animal models such as liver cancer, gastric cancer and S180, further screening and eliminating those with no stable effect, further screening and forming XZ-C immunomodulatory anti-cancer or cancer suppressing Chinese medicine.

It can protect Thymus and increase immune function, protect the bone marrow and increase production of blood, and improve the immune function.

Based on the successful screening of animal experiments, they were applied to clinical practice.

After 10 years of clinical verification of a large number of cases, XZ-C immunomodulatory Chinese medicine can improve the quality of life of patients with advanced cancer, increase immune function, enhance physical fitness, increase appetite, and prolong survival.

2. Experimental Study of Fuzheng Peiben Chinese Medicine on Tumor Inhibition and Immunity Improvement in S_{180}-bearing Mice

(1). Purpose

Through more than 40 years of research and practice in the prevention and treatment of malignant tumors with integrated Chinese and Western medicine in my country, it has been found that many Chinese medicines do have certain effects on the treatment of tumors; in particular, the research on the treatment of malignant tumors with traditional Chinese medicines that have the effect of strengthening the body and strengthening the body, improve human immune function, improve the quality of life and prolong survival.

But TCM treatment of tumors is mostly based on clinical experience observation, and no experimental research.

In order to explore whether the Chinese medicine for strengthening the spleen, nourishing qi and nourishing blood and nourishing the kidney in the traditional Chinese medicine can inhibit tumor growth, the following experiments were carried out.

(2). Method:

1)). Experimental animals:

160 Kunming mice, 5-6 weeks old, weighing 27±2.0g, half male and half male.

2)). **Tumor-bearing animal model:**

The S_{180} ascites tumor strain was respectively inoculated into the axilla of the right forelimb of each experimental mouse according to $1 \times 10^7 \times 0.2$ml tumor cell liquid.

3)). **The experimental grouping.**

It is to randomly divide the experimental animals into

Group A: Buzhong Yiqi treatment group (n=20):

Group B: Qi and blood double tonic treatment group (n=20);

Group C; Nourishing Kidney Yin Treatment Group ((n=20);

Group D: Warming and nourishing kidney-yang treatment group (n=20);

E group: ATCA mixture treatment group (n=20);

Group F: Xiaochaihu Decoction treatment group (n=20);

Group G: Compound capsule treatment group (n=20);

Group H: tumor-bearing control group (n=20)

On the second day after inoculation, each group was given Chinese herbal medicine 0.4ml/(per animal ·d). The tumor-bearing control group was treated with the same amount of normal saline.

4)). **Preparation of Chinese medicines in each group**

According to the original formula, it is made by decoction and concentration, and the concentration of crude drug is 200%.

The above drug concentration and intragastric dose are obtained after replacing the normal human dose with the mouse dose.

In this experiment, Chinese medicines such as the buzhong and invigorating qi, strengthening both qi and blood, nourishing kidney yin, warming support and nourishing kidney yang, combining attacking and support or tonic by applying ATCA mixture, Xiao Chaihu decoction and compound capsules were used to treat S180 mice.

5)). **Observation items:**

The appearance time of tumors and survival time in each group of mice were systematically observed, and their serum protein content, peripheral blood T lymphocyte count and immune organ weight were determined.

(3). Results

Fuzheng Peimu and the ATCA mixture with Fuzheng Peiben as the main component can significantly delay the time of tumor inoculation in mice and inhibit tumor growth (A, B, C, D, E group tumor inhibition rates were 40%, 45%, 44. 5%, 31% and 36%), prolong the survival time of tumor-bearing mice ((A, B, C, D, E group prolonged survival was 27.6%, 45%, 38.5%, 25% and 26.5% respectively)).

The Xiaochaihu decoction mainly based on Quxie, compound capsules can not significantly inhibit tumor growth and prolong survival (compared to group E, $P > 0.05$).

The content of serum protein in groups A, B, C, D, and E increased, A / G ratio increased, peripheral blood T-lymphocyte count increased (compared with G group $P < 0.05$, B, C groups $P < 0.01$), thymus atrophy was significantly inhibited.

(4). Conclusion

This study shows that Fuzheng Peiben or Fuzheng Peiben as the main Chinese medicine treatment can inhibit tumors and enhance immunity, and can increase the level of peripheral blood T lymphocytes to varying degrees, which is more effective than the treatment based on Quxie.

(5). Discuss

1)). The anti-tumor effect and prolonging survival effect of Fuzheng Peiben Chinese Medicine Treatment

In clinical setting, many cancer patients can show symptoms of "deficiency" clinically, such as deficiency of Qi, deficiency of blood, deficiency of Yin, deficiency of Yang, etc.

The treatment should be treated with Fuzheng Peiben Chinese medicine.

This experiment explored the various methods of strengthening the body rightness and supporting the body inside and the anti-tumor effect of both attack and supplement.

The results show that:

Fuzheng Peiben Chinese medicines such as Buzhong Yiqi, Qi and blood double tonic, nourishing kidney yin temperature and kidney yang, and ATCA mixture based on Fuzheng Peiben treatment can significantly delay the time of tumor inoculation in mice, inhibit tumor growth and prolong Survival period of tumor-bearing mice.

a. *From the analysis of tumor inhibition rate of each group as the following:*

In the experimental group of Qi and Blood Double Tonic, its tumor inhibition rate reached 45%;

In the experimental group of nourishing kidney yin, its tumor inhibition rate reached 44.5%,

The second is Buzhong Yiqi, whose tumor suppressing effect is up to 40%, and the effect is also good:

Again, the tumor inhibition rate of the ATCA mixture reached 36%:

However, the effect of the treatment group in the warming supplement for kidney yang is poor, and the tumor inhibition rate is 31%.

It seems that in terms of suppressing tumors it is advisable to adopt the treatment of qi and blood tonic and nourishing kidney yin.

b. *From the analysis from the prolonged survival rate it is as the following:*

The qi and blood supplement group reached 45%, which was the longest group for prolonging survival;

Followed by the nourishing kidney yin group, reaching 38.5%, the effect is also good,

As for the treatment group of ATCA mixture of nourishing middle energy and nourishing qi, warming and nourishing kidney-yang, and combining attack and nourishment, it can also prolong survival, but it is not as good as the treatment group of nourishing qi and blood and nourishing kidney-yin.

The Xiao Chaihu Decoction and compound capsule treatment group, which mainly eliminates evils, showed that it could not significantly inhibit the tumor or prolong the survival period of tumor-bearing mice, and its effect was the worst.

Therefore, from the aspect of prolonging the survival period, the treatment of qi and blood double tonic and nourishing kidney yin is the first choice, followed by the treatment of nourishing the middle and nourishing qi, warming supplement for the kidney yang, and combining the attacking and supplement together.

In terms of both inhibiting tumor and prolonging survival time, the best way to supplement Qi and blood, followed by nourishing kidney-yin, and then supplementing Zhongyiqi and ATCA mixture, the therapeutic effect of warming and nourishing kidney-yang is not obvious.

As for Xiaochaihu Decoction and Compound Capsules, which mainly dispel evil, there is no obvious effect from the results of this experiment.

In a word, all treatments based on Fuzheng culture and the treatment based on Fuzheng culture have the effect of inhibiting tumor growth and prolonging survival to varying degrees, while the treatment based on eliminating pathogens has no obvious effect of inhibiting tumor and prolonging survival.

This experiment shows that: Fuzheng Peiben Chinese medicine or treatment based on Fuzheng Peiben Chinese medicine has obvious anti-tumor effect on smaller tumors, and can significantly extend the survival period and improve the quality of life.

Therefore, it is often used as one of the adjuvant treatments of postoperative radiotherapy and chemotherapy.

Many literatures reported that the clinical use of Fuzheng Peiben to treat malignant tumors has achieved good results.

The results of this experiment further confirmed that the treatment of qi and blood supplementing, nourishing kidney yin, and nourishing middle energy .and qi can inhibit tumors and prolong survival.

These results provide experimental basis for clinical treatment of malignant tumors with integrated traditional Chinese and western medicine.

2)). Fuzheng Peiben Chinese medicine treatment enhances the immune function of the body.

a. **This experiment shows that both Fuzheng Peiben Chinese medicine and treatments based on Fuzheng Pei Ben can increase the level of peripheral blood T lymphocytes to varying degrees.**

For example, at the 4th week, the T lymphocyte levels are as follows:

41. 5% of Buzhong Yiqi group,

44.8% in the qi and blood supplement group,

38.6% in the nourishing kidney yin group,

37.5% of the warming and nourishing kidney-yang group,

35.6% of ATCA mixture group;

b. ***Inhibition of thymic atrophy, such as in the second week***, the thymus index of the treatment group of nourishing middle and nourishing qi, nourishing qi and blood, nourishing kidney yin, warming kidney and strengthening yang, and ATCA mixture were significantly different from the tumor-bearing control group.

It is suggested that the anti-tumor effect of Fuzheng Peiben may be related to the enhancement of the body's immune function.

Some people think that many plant polysaccharides have immunomodulator (immunenoclulator) properties, which are called anti-tumor polysaccharides.

These polysaccharides cannot directly kill cancer cells, but it can activate the body's immune system to release cytokines with anti-tumor effects or enhance the killing effect of LAK cells on cancer cells.

The medications of Fuzheng Pei or strengthening the body and supporting the rightness include plenty of plant polysaccharides,

c. **As reported by Zhao Kesheng:**

Xxxx were extracted, and it was found that the components with a molecular weight of 20,000-25,000 can significantly promote the secretion of tumor necrosis factor (TNF) in vitro by peripheral blood mononuclear cells (PBMC) of normal people and tumor patients.

d. **Chen Kai and others reported:**

The traditional Chinese medicine compound Fuzheng Anti-tumor Liquid can promote the activity of natural killer cells and interleukin-2 (IL-2) of transplanted tumor S180 mice, and can promote the activation of T lymphocytes, Promote the phagocytic function of peritoneal macrophages and increase the weight of spleen and thymus.

In short, the effect of Fuzheng Peiben on the human immune system is very complicated, and further observation and research are needed.

3)). *Fuzheng Peiben traditional Chinese medicine treatment can enhance the body's ability to resist diseases, enhance blood cells and enhance physical strength*

This experiment shows:

Fuzheng Pei medicine can increase the serum protein content of tumor-bearing mice and increase the serum/globulin ratio.

The clinical observation data of our oncology specialist clinic showed that XZ-C4 immunoregulation, anti-cancer and promotion Chinese medicine based on Fuzheng Peiben was used after liver cancer, esophageal cancer, gastric cancer, and colorectal cancer.

Both red blood cells and hemoglobin were higher than the control group, and the reduction of white blood cells was also suppressed.

It shows that the instinct of strengthening the body can improve blood cells and protein, strengthen physical strength, and improve disease resistance.

Fuzheng Peiben has been widely used clinically as one of the treatments of combined Chinese and Western medicine to treat tumors.

The results of this experiment show:

Fuzheng Peiben drug treatment can delay the appearance of swollen scars in inoculated mice, inhibit tumor growth, prolong tumor-bearing survival, enhance the body's immune function and disease resistance, and improve the quality of life. It can provide experimental evidence for clinical Chinese medicine to fight cancer.

3. Immune effect of Chinese herbal medicine on patients with advanced tumors

Most patients with advanced tumors have deficiency syndrome, and the common immune function is low.

The medications of supplement of deficiency and supporting Tonic drugs can enhance the immune function of the body, which is of great significance for the prevention and treatment of tumor patients with low immune function.

1). **Enhance non-specific immune function**

(1)) It can stimulate the thymus and spleen, the immune organs of animals, and increase their weight:

For example, xxxx soup can increase the weight of the thymus of young mice, which is 2.2 times that of the control group.

(2)) Enhance the phagocytic function of macrophages:

Such as xxxx, xxxxxx, xxxxx, xxxxx, xxxxx, etc. can promote the phagocytic function of macrophages, especially the effect of qi medicine is obvious.

(3)) Increase the number of peripheral white blood cells;

Such as xxxx, xxxx, xxxx, xxxxx, xxxxx, etc., can significantly increase the number of white blood cells.

2). *Enhance cellular immune function*

(1) Promote the proliferation of splenic lymphocytes;

For example, xxx **can** increase the number of lymphocytes, and **yam and mulberry** or **Taxillus chinensiscan** increase the proportion of T cells in the peripheral blood.

(2) Improve the conversion rate of lymphocytes:

Many tonic drugs such as xxxxx etc, all have the effect of increasing the conversion rate of lymphocytes.

(3) Enhance red blood cell immune function:

For example, XXXX *and Lycium barbarum* can significantly increase the mouse red blood cell C36 receptor (RBC-C36) rosette rate and red blood cell-immune complex (RBC-IC) rosette formation rate.

3). *Enhance humoral immunity*

(1) Promote antibody production:

For example, XXXX**, etc.** can promote the production of antibodies and increase serum IgG, lgA, lgM and other antibody levels to varying degrees.

(2) Increase the number of spleen antibody-forming cells:

Epidemic stubble polysaccharide injection can increase mouse spleen and cell antibody production by more than 1 time.

Yam polysaccharide can significantly increase mouse spleen and hemolytic plaque forming cells.

However, certain tonic drugs have a dual effect of immune enhancement and suppression.

4. **The enhancement of immune function in the tumor-bearing body by Chinese herbal medicine**

Traditional Chinese medicine believes that the formation and development of tumors are caused by the lack of righteousness in the body, and that the deficiency of righteousness is accompanied by the whole process of tumor occurrence, development, treatment and prognosis.

<u>Fuzheng Peiben is the basic law of traditional Chinese medicine to prevent and treat tumors, and the most prominent is the regulation of the body's immune function, especially the cellular immune function.</u>

Modern studies have proved that the occurrence, development and prognosis of cancer are closely related to the cellular immune status of the tumor-bearing body.

The immune function of tumor patients is suppressed and the body is in an immunosuppressed state.

This phenomenon of immunosuppression is especially obvious in patients with intermediate and advanced stages or patients who have undergone long-term chemotherapy or radiotherapy.

Surgery, radiotherapy, and chemotherapy can cause the body's immune function to decline or become imbalanced.

It is to strengthen the body's immune function through strengthening the body by Chinese medicine, thereby it is to improve the body's anti-cancer ability, improve the effects of surgery, radiotherapy, and chemotherapy, improve the quality of life of patients, and prolong the survival of patients.

1). The effect of Chinese herbal medicine on immune organs

From the drug experiments of protecting immune organs and increasing the weight of immune organs it was found that:

(1) Use the whole XXXX extract 15g/kg, 30g/kg and XXXX or ferula suspension 12.5mg/kg and 25mg/kg for 7 consecutive days can significantly increase the weight of mice spleen and thymus.

(2) Fulfilling mice with 6g/(kg·d) decoction of XXXX or XXX for 7 days can significantly increase the weight of mouse thymus.

It can also antagonize the weight loss of immune organs caused by prednisolone.

(3) Injecting 3Zmg/(kg·d) of XXXX into the mice's abdominal cavity for 7 days can significantly increase the weight of the thymus.

(4) Feeding mice with XXXX Decoction can significantly increase the weight of mice spleen and thymus.

However, it must be noted that there are some Chinese medicines that can reduce the weight of immune organs and promote the shrinkage of immune organs, such as Tripterygium wilfordii, cicada slough, typhus typhus, tumefaciens, rhubarb, etc..

The normal mice are given 0.5g/d rhubarb decoction for the continuous 8 days, which can make the mouse thymus atrophy, the thymus cortex becomes thinner, the cells are obviously reduced, the weight of the spleen is obviously reduced, the lymphocytes (mainly T lymphocytes) around the central artery sheath of the spleen are reduced. And the mice are perfused with 10mg/kg per day continuously for 10 days, which has no obvious effect on the immune organs of mice.

Generally, small doses have no effect, while large doses show a downward trend.

2). Enhancement of Chinese herbal medicine on the function of mononuclear phagocyte system

Chinese medicine polysaccharides, glycosides and many other components can enhance the mononuclear phagocyte system, especially the activity of macrophages, and enhance its immune function.

The anti-tumor effect of macrophages is to activate T cells to release specific macrophages through tumor antigens, and activate macrophages to specifically kill tumor cells:

Through macrophage-mediated cytotoxicity, it kills tumor cells. For example, activated macrophages secrete tumor necrosis factor (TNF), proteolytic enzyme, interferon (IFN), etc. to directly kill or inhibit tumor cell growth.

(1) Lycium barbarum polysaccharide (LBP):

a. **Wang Ling et al. (1995) reviewed the research status of LBP immunomodulation in the second issue of Shanghai Journal of Immunology:**

Gavage of LBP 0.125 (kg· d) mice for 5 consecutive days can improve the phagocytic function of macrophages. It is believed that LBP has a certain immune-promoting effect.

b. **Zhang Yongxiang and others studied the activity of LBP on mouse peritoneal macrophages to inhibit tumor cell proliferation.**

(2) Antler polysaccharide (PAPS):

It can significantly improve the phagocytic function of macrophages in immunocompromised mice caused by hydrocortisone. It has a promoting effect at a concentration of 0.01ug/ml, and has an obvious dose-effect relationship. The most effective PAPS concentration is 1ug/ml.

(3) The total saponins of guttata:

Giving normal mice 300 mg (kg·d) of total saponins of pentaphyllum pentaphyllum, once a day for 7 days, can significantly enhance the ability of peritoneal macrophages to phagocytic cells.

Shou Zhi et al. (1990) reported in the "Journal of Wenzhou Medical College" Volume 20, Issue 1, that Kunming mice were fed 50mg of Penguinum infusion (containing 1.21% of total saponin) daily, 1 day Second, 1 month later, the volume of loose connective tissue and alveolar macrophages under the abdominal wall increased, and the phagocytosis and digestion ability increased.

(4) Achyranthes bidentata polysaccharide:

It can induce macrophages to synthesize IL-1 and secrete tumor necrosis factor-a (TNF-a). Achyranthes bidentata polysaccharide 25mg/kg or 50mg/kg, intraperitoneal injection, can increase the production of IL-1 induced by LPS.

100mg/kg, intraperitoneal injection, can promote the production of TNF-a, and its strength is equivalent to that of BCG.

(5) XXXX:

Using the carcinogen acetamide to cause lung cancer in mice, intraperitoneal administration of psoralen 1mg/20g body weight for 10 days can significantly enhance the phagocytic function of peritoneal macrophages in lung cancer mice.

3). Chinese herbal medicine enhances the immune function of T cells

T cells are extremely important human immune cells in the body, which not only cause specific cellular immunity, but also participate in immune regulation and other functions.

Tumor cells are often accompanied by changes in cell surface antigens. Due to the immune surveillance effect of T cells, T cells sensitized by tumor antigens directly or indirectly kill swelling and pain cells through direct killing effects and the release of cytokines.

(1) Xianling Spleen Polysaccharide (EPS):

Using EPS100mg/ (kg·d) for 5 consecutive days, subcutaneous injection, significantly increased the number of peripheral WBC and T lymphocytes.

(2) Alfalfa polysaccharides (MPS):

It can enhance the proliferation of lymphocytes induced by PHA, CONA, LPS and Pokeweed (PWM) in vitro. MPS 125rng/(kg·d) and 250mg/(kg·d), intraperitoneal injection, the spleen lymphocyte index and lymphocyte number were significantly increased. Intraperitoneal injection of MPS can also partially antagonize the effect of cyclophosphamide in reducing lymphocytes.

(3) Lycium barbarum polysaccharide (LBP):

It can significantly increase the percentage of peripheral T lymphocytes in mice. LBP 5mg/kg·d) intraperitoneal injection for 7 days continuously increased the number of peripheral blood lymphocytes, which was 65.4% in the control group and 81.6% in the administration group, but increasing the dose did not continue to improve this effect.

Under the conditions of T lymphocyte mitogen CONA induction, a small dose of LBP (5-10 mg/kg) can also cause lymphocyte proliferation, indicating that LBP can significantly promote the proliferation of T cells.

(4) <u>Moutan bark</u>:

Gavage at doses of 12. 5g/kg and 25g/kg can significantly improve the transformation function of T Lymba cells in mice.

Red peony:

Gavage at a dose of 25g/han can significantly increase IL-2 activity in mice.

XXXX:

Pushing the stomach at doses of 12.5 g/kg and 25 g/kg can not only significantly improve the T lymphocyte transformation function of mice, but also significantly increase the IL-2 activity of mice at a dose of 25 g/kg.

However, it must be noted that Chinese herbal medicines also have inhibitory effects on T cell immune function, such as Sophora flavescens, Turmeric, Tripterygium serrata, Caulis Spatholobi, Rhubarb, etc. These Chinese medicines that reduce T cell immune function must be used with caution.

4). **The effect of traditional Chinese medicine on LAK cells**

(1) Fangfeng polysaccharide can significantly increase the IL-2 induced killing activity of LAK cells within a certain concentration range.

(2) Seabuckthorn has the effect of promoting blood circulation and removing blood stasis. Injecting seabuckthorn juice (3g/kg) into the abdominal cavity of tumor-bearing mice can significantly increase the NK and LAK activities of their spleen cells.

(3) Cao Wenguang et al. injected C57BL/6 mice intraperitoneally with APS, PAS, and LEP at 5-10 mg/kg, respectively, and found that the three traditional Chinese medicine polysaccharides can significantly promote the proliferation of mouse splenocytes.

Spleen cells were induced in vitro with 225-1000 U/ml rIL-2 at 2 X 106/ml for 4 days, and it was found that the LAK activity of splenocytes in the APS injection group was 70%-120% higher than that in the NS injection group:

The PAS injection group increased by 20%--90%;

The LBP injection group increased by 26%-80%.

(4) From February 1992 to November 1993, Cao Wenguang and others used traditional Chinese medicine LBP combined with LAK and IL-2 to treat 79

patients with advanced malignant tumors that were ineffective in radiotherapy and chemotherapy.

LBP oral dose 1, 7mg/kg, the total amount of LAK application is 1.2-32X 1010, and the total amount of IL-2 application is $3.4-4. 8x10^7U$/person.

The specific plan is to give LBP one month after conventional therapy is stopped, and riL-2 is injected three weeks later, and LBP is given after 4 weeks, a large number of patients' autologous PBL were isolated to induce LAK cells in vitro, and after passing various tests, they were reinfused, and then LBP and IL-2 were given again for 1 week.

The results are as the following:

Among 75 evaluable patients, the efficacy of LAK/IL-2 combined with LBP group (36.36%) was better than that of LAK/IL-2 group alone (18%).

The former combined with LBP group had NK of PBL before and after treatment.

The increase in LAK activity induced by 500U/ml IL-2 in vitro was significantly higher than the latter in the LAK/IL-2 group alone.

It shows that LBP can significantly promote the anti-tumor activity of NK and LAK cells.

Recipes for strengthening the spleen, warming yang, tonifying kidney, replenishing qi, and nourishing yin all have the effect of enhancing LAK activity in the body.

5). __The regulation for Immune Function of Red Blood Cell by Chinese Medicine__

In 1981, American scholar Siegel et al., based on the fact that red blood cells have **immune adhesion** and **type I complement variants (CR1)** on the surface of red blood cells, which can be combined with immune complexes (IC), etc., proposed the concept of "**red blood cell immunity**", clarifying that red blood cells not only have breathing Function, and participate in a variety of immunity and immune regulation of the body, **Such as**

    a. *It is clearing immune complexes in the blood circulation;*

    b. *It is promoting phagocytosis;*

  c. *And it regulates and controls the immune function of lymphocytes;*

  d. *Red blood cells are involved in the production of IFN-y, IL-2, antibodies;*

  e. *It is involved in the regulation and control of immune activity of natural killer cells (NK cells), lymphokine-activated killer cells (LAK cells) and phagocytes.*

1)). The experiments have found that XXXX **(APS)** can enhance the C2bR activity of red blood cells and the function of immune adhesion to tumor cells in cancer patients after acting on the red blood cells of malignant tumors in vitro.

APS can significantly improve the red blood cell immune function of cancer patients.

2)). The Ehrlich ascites cancer mice were treated with **Kuolougen** and compared with the untreated group.

It was found that the RBC-C3bR rosette rate of the untreated group was significantly lower than that of the normal group, and the RBC-C3bR rosette rate of the treated group was significantly higher than that of the untreated group.

And it was slightly higher than the normal group, indicating that the activity of RBC-C3 bR in tumor-bearing mice was significantly decreased, and Kuo Lou Gen could significantly increase the activity of RBC-C3 bR.

A. *The effect of XXXXX on SOD activity of erythrocyte membrane in tumor-bearing mice:*

a. 11 days after the experimental mice were inoculated with cancer cells, the red blood cell SOD activity of **the treated group** was significantly higher than that of the untreated group and the normal group.

b. The SOD of the red blood cell membrane of the tumor-bearing mice decreased significantly in the late stage.

c. This experiment shows that the traditional Chinese medicine **Yaohuafen (Kuolougen)** can restore and enhance the SOD activity of the red blood cells.

B. *The influence of Kuo Lou Gen on the ability of red blood cell immune adhesion to tumor cells:*

Using Ehrlich's ascites cancer cells as target cells, the effect of Kuo Lou Gen on the ability of red blood cells to adhere to tumor cells in experimental mice was measured.

It was found that 11 days after tumor cells were squeezed, the tumor red blood cell rosette rate of untreated mice was (11. 5. 00)%, which is significantly lower than that of normal mice (22.13±6.28)%; while the tumor red blood cell rosette rate of mice in the treatment group (26.54±7.27)% is slightly higher than that of the normal group and significantly higher than that of the untreated group.

C. *The influence of Kuo Lougen on the red blood cell immunity of tumor patients:*

It also significantly enhances the ability of tumor patients' red blood cells to adsorb tumor cells. Laboratory tests found that it has the effect of directly enhancing the rate of RBC-C3bR rosettes in cancer patients, which is significantly different from the normal saline (NS) control group, and the promotion effect is positively correlated with the dose.

5. *Biological Response Modulation (BRMS) of Chinese Medicine and Its Components*

1). A very important feature of Chinese medicine is that it **has a two-way regulation effect** on biological therapy, which can restore the body's immune function to the normal direction or to be balance.

In 1983, Jin Jianping discovered that Astragalus could significantly increase the ability of IL-2 in "spleen deficiency" model mice, but it had no effect on normal mice.

In 1991, when Xiong Xiaoling and others studied the effects of Chinese medicine of chicken blood knee, wintergreen seed, and psoralen on the production of IL-2 in mouse spleen cell blood, It was found that these drugs showed increased, suppressed and no effect on the three groups of immunocompromised, hyperactive, and normal groups, **respectively, reflecting the two-way effect of Chinese medicine.**

2). *In addition, the effect of traditional Chinese medicine on the body is closely related to its dosage.*

a. **Lycium barbarum polysaccharides** can promote IL-2 secretion at low concentrations, but high concentrations can inhibit IL-2 levels.

b. The total concentration of **Paeonia lactiflora** can increase IL-2 production in a dose-dependent manner when the concentration is low, and inhibit IL-2 secretion when the concentration exceeds 12.5 mg.

3). Traditional Chinese medicine preparations have been used in my country for thousands of years, and there are many BRMS options for Chinese medicine.

There are bright prospects for research on anti-cancer immune preparations in this field.

4). *Oral adverse reactions of traditional Chinese medicine preparations are mild.*

5). *Compared with genetic engineering BRMS and exogenous IL-2, IFN, TNF, the advantage of traditional Chinese medicine BRMS is that:*

a. It acts on the systemic immune and anti-cancer system.

b. It can be administered repeatedly without toxic side effects, and can be used for tumors and low immune function caused by chemotherapy and radiotherapy.

c. It promotes the activation of immune cells, releases endogenous cytokines, and inhibits tumor growth.

6). *In modern cancer therapy, Chinese medicine can play a role in at least three aspects:*

① *It Improves the function of the body's inherent anti-cancer organization members, and enhance the body's anti-cancer system (NK cells, TK cells, LAK cytokines);*

② *Certain Chinese medicines have direct anti-cancer effects;*

③ *Some traditional Chinese medicine ingredients can reduce the side effects of radiotherapy and chemotherapy, reduce the degree of leukocyte suppression, accelerate recovery, and even increase the anticancer efficacy of radiotherapy and chemotherapy.*

18

Anticancer effect of cellular immunity

As we all know, the occurrence and development of cancer and the prognosis of treatment are determined by the comparison of two factors:

That is, the biological characteristics of cancer cells and the host's ability to control cancer cells;

If the two are balanced, the cancer is controlled;

If the two are out of balance, the cancer develops.

The biological characteristics and biological behaviors of cancer cells have been briefly described in the previous chapters of this book.

Under normal circumstances, the host's body itself has certain restraining and defensive abilities against cancer cells, but these restraining and defensive abilities are inhibited and damaged to varying degrees when the patients are suffering from cancer, which leads to that cancer cells lose immune surveillance and immune escape of cancer cells occurs, which makes cancer cells metastasize.

1. *Human anti-cancer institutions and their influencing factors*

The human body has a complete anti-cancer immune system: namely

a. *Anti-cancer immune cell series;*

b. *Anti-cancer factor series;*

c. *Humoral immunity series;*

d. *Anti-cancer gene series.*

The body's anti-tumor immunological mechanism can be divided into:

a. **Cellular immunity:**

including T lymphocytes; NK natural killer cells;K cell; LAK cells;

Mononuclear macrophages and so on.

b. **Humoral immunity:**

contains B cells; antibodies against tumors.

c. **Cytokines:**

There are interleukin cell series; IFN; TNF; CSF and so on.

The above-mentioned inherent anti-cancer system and immune substances in the human body are their own substances in the organism. How to mobilize, activate and enhance their regulation effect of anti-tumor biological response occupies an extremely important position and broad prospects in anti-cancer and anti-metastasis treatment.

Therefore, we need to study which <u>anti-cancer cells</u>, which <u>anti-cancer factors</u>, and which <u>humoral immunity</u> can be activated in the human body to strengthen the anti-cancer metastasis.

Here we first review the most impressive achievements of biological therapy in the history of cancer treatment in the 20th century.

1. In the 1930s, Willam Coley and his successor Coley nauts used "Coley toxin" to treat those untreatable advanced cancers.

Among the more than 200 patients with various cancers that can be analyzed, more than 30 have been cured and have lived for more than 30 years.

2. In the early 1980s, Guesada et al. used IFN-a to treat hairy cell leukemia, and the treatment efficiency (CR+PR) reached more than 90%.

3. In the mid-1980s, Rosenberg et al. used LAK/IL-2 to treat patients with advanced metastatic cancer who were ineffective with other existing methods.

Some patients had partial remission (42/228 cases) and complete remission (9/228 cases).

"Biotherapy" is also known as "bioregulator therapy", the "anti-cancer mechanism" in humans and organisms is quite complex. It is a very large network system in terms of structure and function. Under this large system, a "network system" is formed by many members.

In recent years, due to the rapid development of molecular biology, molecular immunology, molecular immunopharmacology, and genetic engineering, the basic and clinical research at the molecular level of "anti-cancer institutions" has been continuously expanded and deepened, and its anti-cancer and anti-metastasis prospects are very attractive.

At present, the research on immunotherapy of anti-cancer molecular biology is mainly concentrated on the "4 subsystems" of the "anti-cancer institution", namely:

(1) "anti-cancer cell therapy",

(2) "anti-cancer cytokine therapy",

(3) "anti-cancer gene therapy",

and (4) "anti-cancer antibody therapy".

The basic characteristics of these molecular biology and molecular immunotherapy are:

a. *The preparations used in molecular biological immunotherapy are "self-substances" in the organism,*

b. *The fundamental difference between it and radiotherapy and chemotherapy is:*

It not only has no progressive damage to the normal tissue cells of the body, especially the cells and functions of the immune system and the structure and function of the bone marrow hematopoietic system, but also mainly has immune response regulation and enhancement effects.

As we all know, radiotherapy and chemotherapy are completely different from this.

a. Chemotherapy is a non-selective "damaging therapy" that kills both cancer cells and normal cells at the same time.

b. It damages the normal tissue cells of the body, severely damages the bone marrow hematopoietic system and immune structure and function, leading to serious consequences.

Biological therapy is a therapy that stabilizes and balances the life mechanism through the regulation of biological response.

American scholar Oldam (1984) proposed the biological regulation (BRM) theory, and then proposed the concept of tumor biotherapy on this basis.

Immune regulation is also an important life mechanism.

Immune structure and its functions are extremely complex, and its essence lies in keeping the body stable in its internal environment by recognizing itself and rejecting dissidents.

Immune defense, immune surveillance and immune homeostasis are the three basic functional types for the body to identify itself and reject dissidents. From the basic point of view of biological function, immune regulation is also one of the basic theories of biological therapy.

There have always been two different views on the occurrence and development of cancer:

a. One view is that the occurrence and development of tumors are regulated and controlled by many factors in the body, especially the "involuntary process" or "controlled process" regulated and controlled by immune factors. The occurrence and development of tumors are subject to immune surveillance, and cancer cells develop only when they escape immune surveillance.

b. Another view is that the occurrence and development of tumors is an "autonomous process" that is basically not restricted by any defense mechanism of the body. The treatment focuses on the tumor itself, and little attention is paid to the regulation of the body's immune system.

Based on these two different points of view, there are two completely different opinions on the treatment policy.

The second view believes that cancer is an "autonomous process" that is basically not restricted by any defense mechanism of the body. Therefore, its treatment policy advocates that the goal and "target" of treatment is simply to kill cancer cells (regardless of the body's immune status).), the methods used are radiotherapy and chemotherapy.

Cao Guangwen and Du Ping put forward an important concept in their "Modern Cancer Biotherapy", which is about the concept of "anti-cancer institution" as the core basis of cancer biotherapy, see picture as the following.

The "anti-cancer agency" in humans and organisms is a huge network system. At present, the basic and clinical research of anti-cancer institutions is expanding and deepening, and it has an extremely important position and broad prospects in anti-cancer metastasis treatment.

Regarding the network function of anti-cancer institutions, the current research is on the structure and function of cytokine network, and other aspects are less researched. The so-called "cytokine network", in simple terms, refers to certain interrelationships between various cytokines in structure and function.

The schematic diagram of anti-cancer institutions and their influencing factors is as the followings:

A.

Anti-cancer institutions and influencing factors

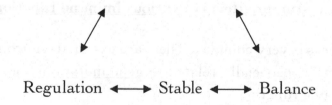

Regulation ⟷ Stable ⟷ Balance

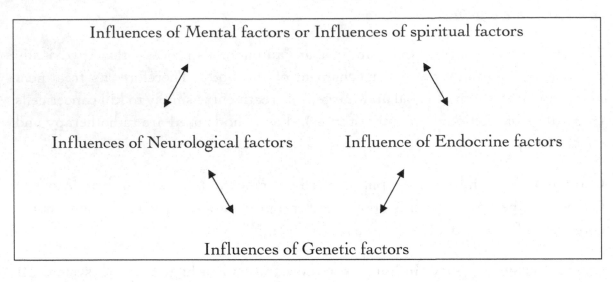

B

Influences of Mental factors or Influences of spiritual factors

Influences of Neurological factors

Influence of Endocrine factors

Influences of Genetic factors

C

Anti-cancer Institutional System

Anti-cancer cell system	Anti-cancer factor system	Anti-cancer gene system
NK cell population	IFN system	Other genes
K cell population	IL2 system	P53 gene
TK cell population	TFN system	Rb gene
LAK cell population	LT system	
Macrophage population	System	
Other cell populations	Other cytokines	
	LT system	

2. Anti-tumor effects of various immune functions

The etiology of tumors is very complex. There are external environmental factors as well as internal factors, especially related <u>to gene mutations, oncogene expression and decreased immune function</u>.

Modern immunology proposes three major functions of the body's immune system:

a. *Immune defense:*

The immune defense function can resist the infection of bacteria, viruses, parasites and other pathogens.

b. *immune stability:*

Immune surveillance function can remove mutant cells and prevent tumors from occurring. If immune surveillance is weak or lose immune surveillance, it can lead to tumors.

c. *immune surveillance.*

The body's immune system is of great significance in anti-tumor. After the normal cells of the body become cancerous, the cells express tumor antigens on the membrane surface, *and the host's immune system recognizes such antigens to generate an immune response; attack and exclude tumor cells.*

The anti-tumor immune response is multi-channel:

a. *Both acquired immune response and natural immune response;*

b. *There are both cellular immune response and humoral immune response;*

c. *Both immune cells and immune molecules participated.*

(1) Anti-tumor effect of cellular immunity

Which anti-cancer immune cells in the human body may be activated and enhanced to stop or resist metastasis of cancer cells?

The immune cells involved in anti-cancer effects in the body are:

1). **Anti-tumor effect of cytotoxic cells:**

  a. Cytotoxic lymphocytes (CTL) play a major role in anti-tumor immunity.

  b. It is a type of anti-tumor lymphocytes with specific killing effect on autologous tumor cells of the same species and restricted by MHC class I and (or) II antigens.

c. Human CTL cells are CD3 and CD8.

d. CTL cells are high in peripheral blood and spleen;

e. Thoracic duct, thymus, bone marrow contain a certain amount;

f. It has strong ability to proliferate in vivo and to accumulate locally in tumors.

g. It is sensitive to radiation;

h. It is sensitive to certain chemotherapy drugs such as cyclophosphamide;

i. CTL is an important effector cell for tumor in situ therapy or for treating tumor in situ.

j. Under certain conditions, it can also produce IL-2, IL-4, IFN, etc.,

k. it activates other anti-cancer immune cells such as killer macrophages, NK cells and killer B cells to play anti-tumor effects together.

In brief, such CTLs have potentially important roles in anti-cancer and anti-metastasis.

2). **Anti-tumor effect of natural killer cells (NK cells)**

a. NK cells are a group of broad-spectrum anti-tumor cells;

b. The killing activity can kill tumor cells without antigen sensitization in advance;

c. It does not rely on antibodies, does not rely on thymus, and is not restricted by MHC.

d. Its main function is to monitor and remove cancerous cells in the human body.

e. Clinical observations have found that people with defective NK cell activity have a significantly higher incidence of malignant tumors.

f. NK cells are an important part of the body's early anti-cancer immune supervision function.

NK cells bind to tumor cells by means of tumor cell receptors on their surface, release perforin (PF) or cytolysin (cylolysin) to puncture the tumor cell membrane, causing cancer cells to flow out and die.

NK cells can release natural killer cell factor (NKCF), which can dissolve tumor cells.

The number of NK cells is small, only equivalent to 3%-5% of lymphocytes, so they have less effect on advanced and larger tumors.

In addition, NK cells can produce IL-2, IFN-y and TNF-a, enhancing the anti-tumor effects of other cells and humoral factors.

The distribution of NK cells in organs and tissues is highest in peripheral blood and spleen, followed by lymph nodes and abdominal cavity cells. There are also NK cells in the alveoli, liver sinusoids, lamina propria of intestinal epithelium, skin and bronchial walls, renal interstitium, esophagus, and genital tract lymphoid tissues. NK cell activity in bone marrow is low, and NK activity cannot be detected in thymus.

NK cells account for 5%-7% of the total number of peripheral blood lymphocytes.

The NK activity of peripheral blood varies greatly among patients. The level of NK activity in vitro is often related to the anticancer effect in vivo.

Therefore, NK activity is often used as an immunological indicator for cancer and to evaluate the strength and prognosis of the body's response to anticancer therapy.

Before the treatment of cancer patients, cancers with reduced or lack of NK activity often develop distant metastases.

Changes in NK activity often parallel the improvement or deterioration of the disease.

In view of the important role of NK cells in anti-tumor immunity, it is very important for biological therapy to find a powerful agent that enhances the anti-tumor activity of NK.

Some microorganisms or their products, such as Bacillus Calmette-Guerin (BCG), Corynebacteriurn Parvwm (CP), and certain cytokines such as IL-2, IFN, immune adjuvants and other interferon inducers can significantly enhance NK activity.

The combined use of IL-2 and IFN-7 result in stronger NK cell activity enhancement than single factor activation.

Multiple cytokines may be of great benefit for enhancing NK activity and eliminating residual cancer cells, reducing metastasis rate and recurrence rate

In addition, the XZ-C immunomodulatory preparations and other traditional Chinese medicines we have developed can activate the effects of NK and IFN-y.

3). K cells

a. There are K cells in human peripheral blood, spleen and abdominal cavity, but not many in thoracic ducts and lymph nodes.

b. The serum of patients with advanced tumors contains a large amount of free tumor antigens. This antigen binds to tumor antibodies, so that K cells cannot bind to tumor cells and therefore cannot play a tumor-killing effect.

c. Removal of free tumor antigens, addition of human anti-tumor antibodies, or use of non-specific immunostimulants can all enhance the activity of K cells.

d. The anti-tumor effect of K cells does not require prior sensitization or complement participation, but requires the presence of anti-tumor antibodies.

__Therefore, K cells are one of the main effector cells for anti-tumor antibody biotherapy.__

4). LAK cells

LAK cells are the most important anti-cancer cell in modern biological therapy.

a. In 1980, Rosenberg and his colleagues discovered that T cell growth factor (TCGF), short-term induction of mouse spleen cells can endow mouse spleen cells with strong tumor activity.

b. Human peripheral monocytes (PBMNC) can significantly kill a variety of human tumor cells under the induction of IL-2 in vitro.

c. In 1982, Grimn called this IL-2 activated cell that can kill NK-resistant tumors as LAK (Lymphokine-activa-ted Killer, LAK) cells.

d. LAK cells are a group of lymphocytes dominated by LGL in morphology.

e. It is activated under the action of IL-2-based cytokines to become powerful anti-tumor cells.

f. It can not only kill tumor cells of the same species, but more importantly, it can kill itself.

g. LAK cells have a broader spectrum of killing tumors than NK cells, that is, LAK cells can kill tumor cells that NK cells cannot.

h. In fact, LAK cells are NK cells activated by IL-2 and T cells that have similar NK cell activity activated by IL-2.

i. From a clinical perspective, any cell activated by IL-2 and other cytokines to become anti-tumor cells can be called LAK cells.

5). Macrophages (Mφ)

Macrophages play an important role in the body's anti-tumor immunity.

a. It is also an effector cell that can dissolve tumor cells.

b. If the patient has obvious macrophage infiltration around the tumor, the tumor spread and metastasis rate is low, and the prognosis is also good.

c. Conversely, if there is less infiltration of macrophages around the tumor tissue, the tumor metastasis rate is high.

d. Prostaglandin E2 can inhibit the secretion of TNF from macrophages at the level of gene transcription, and its antagonist is indomethacin, which can counteract this effect.

6). Anti-tumor effects of monocytes and macrophages

a. In anti-tumor immunity, it not only participates in identifying antigens and presenting antigen information to T cells and B cells, but also participates in killing tumor cells and other antigens.

b. Pathological biopsy tips:

The Patients with high degree of infiltration and which there are a large number of mononuclear-macrophage infiltration around the tumor tissue, especially in primary and metastatic tumors have a lower incidence of tumor spread and metastasis and a better prognosis;

Conversely, where there is no obvious mononuclear-macrophage infiltration in the surrounding tissues of the tumor, the rate of tumor spread and metastasis is high, and the prognosis is poor.

The killing pathways of monocytes and macrophages to tumor cells are non-specific:

(1). Activated mononuclear-macrophages contact tumor cells and directly play a killing effect.

(2). Release cytokines such as TNF and IL-1.

(3). Produce active oxygen, such as H_2O_2.

(4). Release lysosomal enzymes and proteolytic enzymes to kill.

(5). Release arginase. L-arginine is an essential amino acid for tumor cell growth. Monocyte-macrophages release a large amount of arginase after being stimulated to decompose arginine to inhibit tumor growth.

7). Anti-tumor effect of neutrophils

a. A large number of neutrophil aggregation and infiltration can be observed in the surrounding tissues of the tumor. It releases after activation of neutrophils:

    a. **Active oxygen;**

    b. **Fat derivatives;**

    c. **Cytokines, such as IFN, TNF and IL-1;**

These substances have tumor-killing activity.

b. The anti-cancer mechanism of neutrophils:

One is to inhibit tumor growth,

The second is to exert a killing effect.

The killing time takes several hours, which is similar to that of macrophages, but takes longer than lymphocytes and NK cells.

Although the life span of neutrophils is short, but the number is huge, their anti-tumor effect should be paid attention to.

Neutrophils are non-specific killing tumors and have effects on various tumors in the human body.

(2) Anti-tumor effect of humoral immunity

a. *Anti-tumor antibodies can be found in the serum of cancer patients, but not all cancer patients can be detected.*

b. In patients with progressive or metastatic disease, most of the serum antibodies are negative. After surgery or radiotherapy, some patients may turn negative to positive.

c. Anti-tumor antibodies are divided into two types:

Protective and occlusive. The former is beneficial and the latter is harmful.

1)). Protective antibody

The growth and decline of protective anti-tumor antibodies is closely related to tumor dissemination. One month or one week before metastasis, the titer of anti-tumor antibodies in the serum often decreases or turns from positive to negative. There are three types of protective antibodies: cytotoxic antibodies, lymphocyte-dependent antibodies and cytophilic antibodies.

(1) Cytotoxic antibodies:

Such antibodies need to kill tumor cells with the participation of complement, and most of them belong to the 1gM or IgG class.

(2) Lymphocyte dependent antibody (Lymphocyte dependent antibody, LDA):

Most of these antibodies are IgG. After binding to tumor antigens, its Fc fragment binds to the Fc receptors on the surface of lymphocytes, allowing the lymphocytes to adhere to tumor target cells and play a killing effect. Such lymphocytes are antibody-dependent killer cells, namely K cells.

(3) Cytophilic antibodies:

It is an IgG antibody, which is a way for macrophages to specifically kill tumors. It is different from the non-specific killing effect of activated monocyte-macrophage. When cytophilic antibodies are present in body fluids, monocyte-macrophages surround the tumor cells, forming large rosettes.

2)). Blocking factor

There are blocking factors in the serum of animals and tumor patients, which can be proved by experiments.

The blocking factor is closely related to the tumor. After the tumor is removed, the blocking factor disappears. If the tumor recurs, the blocking factor appears.

The blocking factor is specific, it can block autologous or allogeneic tumors of the same type, and has no blocking effect on tumors of different tissue types.

3)). Deblocking factor

After tumor resection, not only the blocking factor disappears from the serum, but also the antagonist of the blocking factor appears in the serum, called unbiocking factor (unbiocking factor), which is also tumor-specific.

(3) Anti-tumor effects of cytokines

Which anti-cancer factors in the human body can be activated and enhanced to resist metastatic cancer cells?

a. Cytokines play an important role in the body's cellular immune response to viruses, parasites, bacteria and cancer.

b. It is used in cancer treatment and bone marrow regeneration in clinical trials.

Therefore, the research on cytokines has increased significantly in the past 10 years, and a large number of papers on the structure, receptors and functions of cytokines have been published.

The following is a brief description of the five major types of cytokines:

a. *interleukin,*

b. *colony stimulating factor,*

c. *tumor necrosis factor,*

d. *interferon,*

e. *and growth factor.*

1). **Interferon (IFN)**

a. In the 1930s, it was discovered that virus-infected cells can protect surrounding cells from virus infection.

b. In 1957, Isaacs and Lindenmann discovered a protein, which is **a protein produced by cells when the cells of the body are damaged or stimulated by a virus**. They call this protein an interferon.

c. In the next few years, people realized that <u>interferon can resist cell differentiation and has immune regulation function.</u>

d. Interferon is a cytokine and has a variety of biological functions. It is now known that interferon is divided into three categories: a, y, ß.

e. <u>IFN-a is mainly derived from white blood cells;</u>

<u>IFN-ß is mainly derived from fiber cells;</u>

<u>IFN-y is mainly derived from T lymphocytes.</u>

f. IFN has anti-proliferative effects on certain tumor cells;

Its anti-cancer effect may be related to its immunomodulatory activity;

It can increase the activity of natural killer cells (NK) and macrophages.

g. <u>**The main preparations of interferon are:**</u>

a. **Drug name Interferon-alfa-2a, trade name Roferon⑧-A;**

b. **The name of the drug is Interferon-alfa--2 b, the name of the drug is Intron⑧-A**

c. **Clinical application of interferon:**

IFN-a is mainly used for

   a). **Hematological tumors and lymphomas:**

For <u>hairy cell leukemia (HCL),</u> <u>chronic myeloid leukemia</u>, <u>primary thrombocytosis,</u> <u>multiple myeloma</u>, <u>non-Hodgkin's lymphoma.</u>

   b). **Solid tumor:**

<u>Kaposi's sarcoma (Kaposi'sarcoma)</u>, <u>renal cell carcinoma</u>, <u>metastatic melanoma.</u>

d. IFN has the effect of slowing down the progression of hematological malignancies and solid tumors. But it is only partial and short-lived.

2). **Interleukins (interleukins, IL)**

a. Interleukins are natural components of the human immune system.

b. They are a type of cellular kinases.

c. The chemical components are proteins. They are a group of molecular families. They mainly act on the signal transmission of the immune system and their main functions are immune regulation and immune modification.

d. The original intent of Interleukin is to signal and transmit between cells in the immune system.

e. **IL is secreted by white blood cells.**

When they bind to receptors on the cell membrane, the target cells are activated.

f. **<u>The complex balance between cell activity and immune regulation is coordinated through the secretion of IL and its effect on the cells of the immune system</u>.**

g. So far, **<u>only IL-2 and IL-11</u>** have been used clinically, and their role in treating tumors and stimulating the production of hematopoietic cells is under clinical observation.

(1) Interleukin-2 (IL-2):

    a.   This lymphocyte line was first described in 1976.

It is a T cell growth factor, mainly produced by activated T helper cells, and has a strong role in regulating the immune function in the body.

    b.   ***Biological activity of IL-2:***

IL-2 is an important substance for the body to produce an immune response. **It has various biological activities**:

Including

① promoting the proliferation of all subpopulations of T cells,

② Increase the activation of cytotoxic T cells, NK cells and monocytes.

③ f.The activation of peripheral blood lymphocytes is called Lymphoblastic Killer Cells (LAK).

④ IL-2 can support the growth of B cells and

⑤ also promote the release of IFN-a, GM-CSF and TNF.

Since 1984, recombinant IL-2 has been tried to treat a variety of malignant tumors.

    c.   There have been many reports of IL-2 alone or in combination with LAK cells in the treatment **of renal cell carcinoma and malignant melanoma.**

In May 1992, the FDA approved IL-2 to treat **adult metastatic renal cell carcinoma.**

Recombinant IL-2 has been used as a single preparation or combined with LAK cells, TIL cells, other biological regulatory factors, chemotherapy, etc. to treat tumors.

(2) Interleukin-4 (IL-4):

IL-4 is mainly produced by activated T cells.

① Effect on B cells:

It can stimulate the growth and differentiation of static B cells, stimulate B cells to replicate DNA, and become a growth factor for B cells.

② Effect on T cells:

It can stimulate the growth of T cells and increase the production of IL-2.

It promotes the proliferation of cytotoxic T cells and activate LAK cells.

IL-4 promotes the growth of TIL and increases the cytotoxic effect on melanoma cells.

Clinical application of IL-4:

The clinical trial of IL-4 has entered Phase II, mainly for renal cell carcinoma, melanoma, chronic lymphocytic leukemia, and Hodgkin's disease.

(3) Interleukin-12 (IL-12):

IL-12 has immunomodulatory and anti-tumor effects, and monocytes are the main source of IL-12.

Its main functions are:

a. It stimulates the proliferation of active T cells and NK cells;

b. It induces T lymphocytes and NK cells to release IFN-y.

Clinical application of IL-12:

The treatment of metastatic renal cell carcinoma and melanoma has completed Phase I and Phase II clinical trials.

3). **Tumor Necrosis Factor (TNF)**

In 1975, Old et al. isolated a substance produced by activated macrophages, monocytes and lymphocytes after exposure to endotoxin, called tumor necrosis factor (TNF).

In 1984, the TNF gene was cloned to make People can obtain large amounts of recombinant TNF.

The biological effects of TNF:

In vitro experiments have shown that the effect of TNF on cells is cytotoxic, and it can affect the microvessels of the tumor, eventually leading to necrosis in the center of the tumor. Especially TNF can induce vascular endothelial cells to express tissue factor to promote cellulose deposition and embolism.

In the anti-tumor effect of TNF, T lymphocytes play an important role. Many observations have proved that TNF and IFN-y have a synergistic anti-tumor effect.

TNF has been tested for the treatment of melanoma, colon cancer, non-small cell lung cancer, ovarian cancer, etc., but **unfortunatel**y it has not shown a definite relief or treatment effect on any kind of cancer.

When TNF is used in combination with IFN-y, IFN-y increases the expression of TNF receptors on the cell surface, so that the effect of TNF on cells is enhanced.

The combination of TNF and IFN-y treats various refractory malignant tumors.

The strategy is that IL-2 can stimulate the activity of cytotoxic lymphocytes, and TNF can expand the effectiveness of anti-tumor.

As a result, the side effects of the two drugs appeared during the entire treatment. Only 1 case of breast cancer and 1 case of renal cell carcinoma were relieved after the combination medication.

4). Hematopoietic Growth Factor (HGF)

HGF was also called clonal stimulating factor in the past, because it can induce the formation of specific cell clones in vitro.

The effect of HGF on normal blood cell production:

Blood cells are differentiated from polyphasic stem cells (PPSC). There are few PPSCs in the bone marrow and they can differentiate into any blood cells.

In the bone marrow, every PPSC divides into two daughter cells, one enters the differentiation pathway, and the other returns to the cell bank to maintain a static state.

PPSC grows and develops in the sinusoid space surrounded by bone marrow stroma.

(1) **Neutrophils:**

It is a type of granular cell, accounting for 50%-70% of the total white blood cell count. It has 6 steps in its maturation process, namely, bone marrow blasts, pre-marrow cells, and bone marrow cells. These 3 steps require 4-5 days, and then no more It undergoes mitosis, but continues to mature for about 6 days before being released into the peripheral blood. Half of the cells circulate freely, and half of the cells adhere to the blood vessel wall. Cells circulating in the blood move to the tissues after 6-8h, where they can live for 2-3d. Usually the number of circulating cells is three times that of the reserve cells in the bone marrow, so there is always a reserve of neutrophils in the body. Once severe damage occurs, the lifespan of a neutrophil will be reduced to several hours.

(2) **Platelets:**

Platelets, also called **thrombocytes.** Its progenitor cells are megakaryocyte clone forming units. In the bone marrow are megakaryocytes, which then differentiate into megakaryocytes, which release multiple platelets. Platelets can form small thrombi that can stop bleeding on the damaged blood vessel wall and activate clotting factors. Platelets can survive in the blood for 7-8 days.

One major function of platelets is to contribute to <u>hemostasis</u>: the process of stopping bleeding at the site of interrupted <u>endothelium</u>.

In addition to their role in coagulation and healing, platelets also act as the immune system's first responders when a virus, bacterium, or allergen enters the bloodstream.

(3) **Lymphocytes:**

Lymphoid stem cells differentiate into pre-T or B lymphocytes.

Pre T lymphocytes mature in the thymus and become prothymocytes, lymphoblasts and T lymphocytes. They can mediate cellular immunity. Can circulate freely in the tissues and peripheral blood. When stimulated by antigens, T cells produce a variety of cytokines to control specific immune responses.

The pre-B lymphocytes gradually mature after moving to the spleen and lymph nodes. When they respond to antigen-antibodies appearing on their cell membranes, they become mature B lymphocytes and finally plasma cells. Plasma cells secrete specific immunoglobulins, namely antibodies, responsible for humoral immunity. B lymphocytes account for 20%-25% of all lymphocytes.

Blood cell growth factor controls the development of blood cells by stimulating the differentiation and maturation of cells.

Granulosa cell cloning stimulating factor (G-CSF) has been tested in preclinical animals. After the use of 5-FU and whole body irradiation, G-CSF can accelerate the recovery of neutrophils. A further study with monkeys showed that intravenous injection of GM-CSF (granulocyte-macrophage cloning stimulating factor) increased white blood cells after 24-72 hours.

Clinical trials began in 1986, and the FDA approved the use of G-CSF in 1991, which can reduce the incidence of infection in patients suffering from bone marrow cancer who receive myelosuppressive chemotherapy.

19

Source background and experience
of scientific research topics

(1) The background of the subject and the completion process (tortuous process)

Three monographs and new books are actually the key scientific and technological projects that I undertook during the "Eighth Five-Year Plan"-project name supervised by the National Science and Technology Commission:

a. **"the Experimental and Clinical Research of further Exploration of Anti-cancer and Anti-cancer Chinese Herbal Medicine against Liver Cancer, Gastric Cancer, and Precancerous Lesions on the Combination of Chinese and Western Anti-metastatic Prevention and Treatment."**

b. The topic name of the special contract of the "Eighth Five-Year" National Science and Technology Research Project:

"Clinical and Experimental Study of Traditional Chinese Medicine and Western Medicine Treating Gastric Cancer and Precancerous Lesions".

In April 1991, the author submitted an application to the National Science and Technology Commission for the key scientific and technological research projects during the "Eighth Five-Year Plan" period. Clinical research".

In June, Director Tian from Hubei Provincial Science and Technology Commission organized three project leaders (1 Tongji Medical College, 1 Hubei Medical College, and 1 Hubei College of Traditional Chinese Medicine) of our province to apply for the National Science and Technology Commission's key project to Beijing The Authority reports.

Two months later, Director Tian of the Provincial Science and Technology Commission went to Beijing with three project leaders to further report the project design and accept the task to the Ministry of Health.

Two months later, the project task was issued. While planning to sign the "Eighth Five-Year National Science and Technology Research Project Special Contract", Professor Xu Ze had a sudden acute myocardial infarction, anterior and high sidewall myocardial infarction. After rescue and treatment, he was hospitalized for half a year and rested for half a year after being discharged. The National Science and Technology Commission's research projects were stranded and suspended.

In 1993, Professor Xu Ze's physical health gradually recovered, and the idea of continuing to study the content of the subject has sprung up.

It is because the author has followed up a large number of patients after radical cancer resection. It was found that recurrence and metastasis after cancer surgery are the key factors affecting the long-term curative effect after radical operation of cancer. It is necessary to study the clinical basis and effective methods to prevent postoperative recurrence and metastasis. It was determined to do some research work that should be done and within his ability in this regard.

But He had ideas but no research funding, so he began to find ways to self-finance research funding.

In 1993, when Dr. Xu's wife retired, she applied for a clinic, and her meager income was used as the starting point for research funding.

It was used to purchase Kunming mice from the Animal Center of the Chinese Academy of Medical Sciences for animal experiments, prepare animal cages and related equipment and instruments for experiments, and start animal experiments. The meager income of the clinic is used to support Professor Xu Ze 's animal research and it was to save application with careful calculation. The six rooms on the second floor are used for animal experiments.

In 1996, Professor Xu Ze was 63 years old and also applied for retirement. Since then, with the support of this meager income, a series of experimental studies and clinical verification have been carried out. After 16 years of hard work, it has basically completed the key tasks of the National Science and Technology Commission, bringing together experimental and clinical research materials, data, and overall results. Successively it has been published three monographs:

① "New Understanding and New Model of Cancer Treatment", written by Xu Ze, published by Hubei Science and Technology Press, January 2001, published by Xinhua Bookstore;

② "New Concepts and New Methods of Cancer Transfer and Treatment", written by Xu Ze, published by People's Military Medical Press, January 2006, issued by Xinhua Bookstore across the country In April 2007, the General Administration of Publication of the People's Republic of China issued the "three hundred" original book certificate.

③ "New Concepts and Methods of Cancer Treatment" by Xu Ze and Xu Jie, published by Beijing People's Military Medical Press in October 2011. Later, American medical doctor Dr. Bin Wu and others translated into English. The English version was published in Washington on March 26, 2013 and distributed internationally.

(2) Some experiences

In the past, the author conducted scientific research in medical colleges with the help of superiors and colleagues. The laboratory conditions are excellent. He has undertaken the projects of the National Natural Science Foundation of China, the National Science and Technology Commission, and the Provincial Science and Technology Commission. He has achieved two scientific research results. The item is the domestic advanced level, and the item is the international advanced level. It has won the second prize of Hubei Provincial Science and Technology Achievements twice and the first prize of Hubei Provincial Health Science and Technology Achievements.

But now it's different. In this special case, how can one proceed and complete national tasks in a clinic or outpatient department, with no conditions and no equipment?

We had the following superficial experience:

1. Self-reliance and self-financing. Outpatient services for patients, and outpatient income as research funding.

2. Keep the outpatient medical records and follow-up throughout.

3. Establish special scientific research collaborations and conduct collaboration and cooperation in accordance with scientific research plans.

4. Establish detailed medical records (including patient's epidemiological data), and analyze in depth the successful experience, failure lessons and the particularity of the disease in each case.

5. Adopt the scientific research cooperation strategy of instrument sharing, equipment sharing, and achievement sharing. Instead of adding large-scale instruments and equipment, collaborate with the affiliated hospital of the Medical College, and the inspection of high-precision instruments and equipment will be conducted in the affiliated hospital of the Medical College.

6. Self-selected scientific frontier topics, failed to declare the topic (because of its rarity in recent years), and only report the results of profit research to the ministry, province and city after the research results.

7. In the private outpatient department of the old professors, through the strategy of scientific research collaboration and sharing of instruments and equipment with colleges and universities, and the results sharing strategy, the full use of the advanced equipment conditions of colleges and universities and their own decades of clinical experience can also be carried out. Complete scientific research projects.

After 20 years of hard work, a series of experimental research and clinical verification work have been carried out.

Finally, it had basically completed the "8th Five-Year" research project of the National Science and Technology Commission that we applied for, and collected experimental and clinical research materials, data, conclusions, and summaries.

The author has written more than 100 scientific research papers. Because there is no research funding, he cannot send the papers to the journal for publication. Instead, he publishes them as a new book. He has published more than 18 monographs.

Now this will be 19th book, and all of these monographs are three different stages of our hard work, difficult climb, step by step, scientific research footprints, three different levels of achievements, and three different peaks.

This is a series of coherent scientific research steps and scientific research processes.

The above briefly describes the background and context of my three monographs and new books:

From the results of a clinical follow-up discovery to experimental tumor research findings;

From the review of clinical medical practice cases to the analysis, evaluation and reflection of postoperative adjuvant chemotherapy cases, the shortcomings of traditional chemotherapy were discovered.

Look for anti-cancer and anti-metastatic new drugs from natural medicines (Chinese medicine), carry out in vitro and in vivo experiments of cancer-bearing models to discover and make xz-c series of immunomodulatory Chinese medicines, and then to clinical verification.

Now 50 years and more than 12,000 cases have been clinically verified and observed.

From experimental basic research and clinical verification observations to a theoretical understanding, a series of innovative theories, some of which are original innovations, proposed a series of reform measures for traditional therapies, and proposed strategies to overcome cancer and strategic prospects.

Such as the above research content and research results, some of which are the original and innovative scientific research papers with intellectual property rights that were first reported in the international are filled in three monographs and published in the form of books.

20

How can I get out of "Shen Gui"?

1. What is Deep boudoir that we are facing?

XZ-C (XU ZE China) immunomodulated anti-cancer and anti-metastatic series of traditional Chinese medicine preparations have been passed through 7 years of animal experiment research.

Over the years, a large number of clinical patients with advanced cancer have been verified by oncology clinics.

The vast majority of patients can improve symptoms and relieve pain, and those with metastases can stabilize or control the disease, improve quality of life, and prolong survival.

__However, it still failed to promote the application__.

A large number of advanced cancer patients in the whole province and the whole country cannot benefit from it.

Many patients with cancer metastasis urgently need anti-metastatic, relapsed XZ-C immunomodulatory drugs, so they should try to promote the transformation of scientific research results.

2. What is the advantages and the details which need to be solved of XZ-C series?

a. XZ-C series of immunomodulatory drugs are the traditionally developed Chinese medicine preparations that our laboratory has undergone long-term cancer-bearing animal experiment screening and long-term clinical application verification and observation, all of which are independent intellectual property rights of original innovation or independent innovation.

b. XZ-Cl-10 series are still:

1). These achievements are still in the deep boudoir and no one knows these achievements.

Or "'Cultivated in the deep girl's unrecognized"

2). How can I get out of "Shen Gui"?

3). There are three main reasons for locking "Boudoir":

① XZ-C$_{1-10}$ has more than 10:

Which one should we develop?

There are 7-8 supplementary treatments such as Xiaoshui Decoction and Tuihuang Decoction.

Which one should we develop?

② To develop one, it needs 3-5 million yuan, and there is no development fund.

③ Pharmaceutical plants that have passed the GMP without investment and development.

We attach importance to the construction of independent intellectual property rights and insist on using our own independent innovation research results in pharmaceuticals and formulations. Now we have 16 series of XZ-C immunomodulatory anti-cancer and anti-metastatic series preparations with independent intellectual property rights. Cancer animal laboratory screening and long-term clinical trials of a large number of patients with advanced cancer patients have shown different degrees of innovation and creation.

They are welcomed by the majority of patients and hope to walk out of the anti-metastatic path with Chinese characteristics.

1. Social benefit assessment:

Cancer is currently a common disease that threatens human life and accounts for the first and second causes of death for urban residents in China. It goes without saying that cancer is still one of the medical problems.

At the beginning of the 21ˢᵗ century, **the most important problem in cancer treatment is metastasis.**

The most urgent problem that needs to be solved at present is how to resist metastasis, but **metastasis is only a phenomenon, an understanding, and an object of research.** It is invisible and untouchable.

How to make this goal of anti-metastasis be concrete, how to clearly understand the specific process, steps and mechanism of cancer cell metastasis?

We propose anti-cancer metastasis as the goal.

In order to achieve this goal, the goal of anti-transfer should be specified, otherwise, the purpose of anti-transfer can not be achieved,

The content of this book proposes 14 new discoveries, new theories, and new concepts.

For the process of cancer cell metastasis, the countermeasures are specific, for example,

1). where the current cancer research problem is mentioned in this book? It's about anti-transfer.

2). it was to discover and propose that cancer manifests in the human body in three forms. This third form is cancer cells in the process of metastasis:

This new understanding and new doctrine initiative will cause a series of changes and updates in the diagnosis and treatment of chain reaction.

3). it was to discover and propose that the goal of cancer treatment should be aimed at these three forms;

4). it was to discover and propose a two-point, one-line theory of the entire process of cancer development, thinking that cancer treatment should not only pay attention to two points, but also should cut off the first line;

5). The specific measures to discover anti-metastasis should be to hunt down and intercept cancer cells in the process of metastasis;

6). It was to discover and advocate new concepts and models for cancer treatment. That is, a new model of immunochemotherapy should be developed;

7). a new model of cancer metastasis treatment should be discovered and proposed,

8). a "three steps" of anti-cancer metastasis treatment should be proposed.

Some of the above new insights, new theoretical insights, new concepts have important academic significance and important academic value, and will have an important impact on the development of oncology medical science, which may benefit thousands of patients with cancer metastasis.

It is to walk out of a new way to overcome cancer.

How to find anti-cancer cell metastasis measures and from which route to explore?

In the research of anti-cancer, Chinese medicine is an advantage of China. It is to develop this advantage in anti-metastasis research, to play the advantages of China, to surpass the international advanced level.

In this book, XZ-C immunomodulates anti-cancer and anti-metastatic traditional Chinese medicines have passed through 3 years of experimental screening of tumor-bearing tumor models in cancer-bearing animal models, and 11 years of clinical verification and application. It not only benefit patients with metastatic cancer, but also has achieved billions of economic benefits for the country.

The Collections and summary of anti-cancer and anti-cancer metastasis research, scientific and technological innovation, scientific research achievements

Part II

(Brief or Short Book)

Technological innovation • Scientific research achievements

Walk out the new path to conquer cancer

XZ-C immunomodulatory anti-cancer therapy has formed

For more than 20 years the new path to conquer cancer has been found

Summary and Collections

The theoretical system of XZ-C immune regulation and control cancer treatment has been formed, and it has been undergoing clinical application and observation verification

TABLE OF CONTENTS

PREFACE

Why did the title of this book be named as "walked out the New Way to Conquer Cancer"?

The origin of the book title is due to the guidance and enlightenment in the letters from several experts, scholars, predecessors and teachers:

1. On July 2th, 2001 in the letter from **Academician Wu Min** it was mentioned:

"The general impression is: *the model from clinical to experimental and from experimental to clinical is very good; it is also very correct to take the path of integrating Chinese and Western medicine. I sincerely wish you to keep moving forward and find a new way to overcome cancer.*"

2. On February 22th, 2006 in Academician Tang Zhaoxian's letter it was mentioned:

"**...Traditional Chinese medicine and biological therapy are the two most promising ways of anti-metastasis,** *especially Chinese medicine and traditional Chinese medication. I hope you will take the path of anti-metastasis with Chinese characteristics.*"

3. In Academician Liu Yunyi's letter on March 22th, 2006 it was mentioned:

"...I very much agreed *with the concepts and thinking you put forward in the book to conquer cancer... I hope you can make a breakthrough contribution in Chinese medicine and traditional Chinese medication so that the majority of patients will benefit, Chinese medicine can be further developed, and it makes my medical career reach world status. Or, it is to benefit the majority of patients, enable the further development of Chinese medicine and traditional Chinese medication, and make our medical career reach the world status.*"

4. In a letter from Academician Wu Xianzhong on January 9th, 2006, it was mentioned:

*"A tumor is a hard bone that it is difficult to be gnawed, and it should continue to be gnawed. Fortunately, everyone is very objective. Only if it is effective or it works, whether it is to treat, to deal with tumors, or the body, or to reduce the reaction of radioactivity and chemotherapy, it will be supported." I*n the letter of April 10th, 2012 it was mentioned: *"...I think the path you have traveled is very distinctive,* which Chinese medicine is innovative in application dosage forms, administration methods, drug combinations, and the development of XZ-C series of drugs, and it has formed its own patent, *and this road should continue*."

Thank them for their guidance, leading, and help to our scientific research work, scientific research thinking, research direction, research route, research goal, and research method. Our research work has been following the direction of their guidance, and I would like to extend my gratitude to academicians such as Wu Hao, Tang Zhaota, Wu Xianzhong, and Liu Yunyi.

In the past 35 years (1985-present) our cancer research has achieved a series of scientific and technological innovation and scientific research results in animal experimental research, clinical basic research, and clinical verification. After 35 years of hard work, the XZ-C immune regulation and control anti-cancer treatment has been formed.

In the past 60 years, a new way to conquer cancer has been walked out.

Over the past 60 years, this series of experimental and clinical research work has been enthusiastically supported and cordially guided by Qiu Fazu, an internationally renowned surgeon and a master of general surgery in my country.

In 1990, when the author submitted to the National Science and Technology Commission for the "Eighth Five-Year Plan" key scientific and technological projects (further explore the anti-cancer and anti-cancer Chinese herbal medicines on liver cancer, gastrointestinal cancer precancerous lesions, anti-cancer, anti-metastasis experimental and clinical research) application, Academician Qiu stated in the expert opinion: *"Research on cancer metastasis and how to prevent it is a very important topic at present. It is feasible to explore clinical prevention and treatment methods through experimental research and it is a work that is beneficial to the people."*

Under the rigorous and scientific style of study and guidance from my teacher, Academician Qiu, we have initially completed the above project work, and I would like to thank you.

Scientific research must be fed by literature. In 1986, we had just established an experimental surgical animal laboratory to create animal models of cancer metastasis and conduct experimental research. We read Professor Gao Jin's book "Invasion and Metastasis of Cancer----—Basic Research and Clinic"; read the monograph "Basic and Clinical of Liver Cancer Metastasis and Recurrence" by Academician Tang Zhaotan. The theories in the two books made us suddenly enlightened, and also encouraged and promoted our experimental work and clinical verification work from another aspect. Professor Tang Zhaotao puts forward in his monograph: ***"The next important goal of primary liver cancer research is prevention and treatment of recurrence and metastasis". And it was said: "Metastasis and recurrence has become a bottleneck to further improve the survival rate of liver cancer, and it is also one of the most important difficulties in overcoming cancer."***

These theoretical documents have given us the wisdom and courage to update our thinking and be creative, and also strengthen the confidence and determination of our experimental team.

I would like to extend my gratitude to Academician Tang Zhaotan and Professor Gao Jin.

In the past 7 years, we have used more than 6000 tumor-bearing animal models to explore basic questions one after another. In vivo anti-tumor experiment screening of 200 kinds of Chinese herbal medicines in tumor-bearing animal models was completed by several graduate students of mine, including Master Zhu Siping, Dr. Zou Shaomin, Master Li Zhengxun, Master Liu Liling, etc. They carried out and completed a large number of arduous and meticulous experimental work. They worked hard, day and night, and made contributions to the development of cancer prevention and anti-cancer experimental oncology medicine. I would like to express my sincere thanks.

1

The theoretical system of XZ-C immune regulation and cancer treatment has been formed, and it has been undergoing clinical application and observation verification

XZ-C new concept for cancer treatment
The brief introduction is as follows:

(1) **The concept of cancer therapy**

The new model believes that healing or curing should be through regulation and control rather than killing:

Summary

1. The new model of cancer believes that:

Cancer cure should be through regulation and control rather than killing. The last step in curing cancer is to mobilize the reappearance of the host's control, rather than destroy the last cancer cells.

Why?

It is because killing can only kill cancer cells in the few days when the medicine is used, it cannot be done once and for all. Afterwards, the division and proliferation, recurrence, progress, and remission are still there. The relief is only temporary. Thereafter it still divides, relapses, progresses, it is only a temporary phenomenon.

2. The traditional concept thinks:

Cancer is the constant division and proliferation of cancer cells, and its treatment goal must be to kill cancer cells. Therefore, the traditional therapeutic concept of cancer is based on killing cancer cells.

---

(2) Cancer etiology and pathogenesis

XZ-C proposed:

Thymus atrophy and weakened immune function may be one of the causes and pathogenesis of cancer

Summary

This book was first proposed internationally <<One of the etiology and pathogenesis of cancer may be thymic atrophy and weakened immune function>> (After checking the novelty: this is the first time in the world to put forward)

Our laboratory found from experimental research results:

The thymus of cancer-bearing mice showed progressive shrinkage, reduced in size, blocked cell proliferation, and decreased mature cells. In the late stage of the tumor, the thymus gland is extremely atrophy and the texture becomes hard. It may be atrophy of the thymus, impaired central immune organ function, low immune function, decreased immune surveillance ability and immune escape.

(3) Theoretical basis and experimental basis for cancer treatment

XZ-C proposed:

The theoretical basis and experimental basis for cancer treatment of <u>"Thymus protection and increase immune function"</u>

Summary

This book first proposed<< *<u>Theoretical Basis and Experimental Basis of the principles of cancer treatment:</u>*

<u>XZ-C Immunomodulation Therapy-----Thymus Protection and Immunity increase (protection of the thymus and increase immunity), and protection of the marrow to produce blood (protection of bone marrow stem cells)>>.</u>

This is the first international proposal.

As the above-mentioned experimental research has found new enlightenment, the treatment principle must be to prevent the progressive atrophy of the thymus, promote the hyperplasia of the thymus, protect the bone marrow hematopoietic function, improve the immune surveillance, and control the immune escape of malignant cells.

Therefore, its treatment should be "thymus protection and increase immunity" to protect the thymus and increase immunity. It is the theoretical basis and experimental basis of XZ-C immunomodulation therapy for "thymus protection and immune function promotion".

(4) Principles of cancer treatment

XZ-C proposes:

To establish a comprehensive treatment view

Summary

This book first put forward *<<the Goal or Target of Cancer Treatment must aim at both the tumor and the host simultaneously or at the same time and the concept and view of the comprehensive treatment should be established >>.*

We suggest that all hospitals around the world should establish a comprehensive view and concept of cancer treatment in radiotherapy and chemotherapy, and reform the current concept of one-sided treatment concept.

No one has ever mentioned the concept of "full treatment view" or "one-sided treatment view" in this article mentioned for the first time in the world.

At present, radiotherapy and chemotherapy in hospitals at home and abroad only kill cancer cells. We think this is a one-sided view of cancer treatment. Not only did it fail to protect the patient's immunity, but it also killed a large number of host immune cells and bone marrow hematopoietic cells, resulting in lower immune function with chemotherapy, and metastasis during chemotherapy.

(5) The model of cancer treatment

XZ-C proposes:

To establish a plan of multidisciplinary comprehensive treatment

Summary

This book is the first international initiative to propose **<<Establishing a plan of multidisciplinary comprehensive treatment >>**

We propose:

The whole course of treatment is the main axis:

> *Mainly surgery + biological treatment, immunomodulation treatment, integrated traditional Chinese and western medicine treatment, XZ-C immunomodulation treatment...*
>
> *Short-term treatment is the secondary axis:*
>
> *Radiotherapy and chemotherapy are the mainstays. Long-term treatment and excessive treatment should not be used. The current long-term treatment status in some hospitals should be changed.*
>
> This new concept of full-course treatment and short-term treatment is proposed in this article for the first time in the world.
>
> At present, various hospitals at home and abroad are mainly radiotherapy and chemotherapy for cancer treatment. The current status of comprehensive treatment in various provinces in my country is based on the three traditional treatments. The results of such comprehensive treatment still have not prevented recurrence and metastasis. As for biological therapy, immunotherapy, differentiation induction therapy, combined Chinese and Western therapy, and immunomodulation therapy, none of them have been included in the oncologist's treatment plan.

(6) Principles of cancer metastasis treatment

The key to cancer treatment is anti-metastasis

> Summary
>
> This book proposes that the key to cancer research is anti-metastasis.
>
> The basic principle of cancer treatment is anti-metastasis. The main feature of the new concept of cancer treatment is to control metastasis.
>
> Metastasis is the main cause of cancer death so that metastasis is the key to cancer treatment.
>
> **The main reason cancer causes such a high mortality rate is metastasis. The original traditional therapy failed to reduce the long-term high mortality rate. The main reason for its failure was the failure to target and control the metastasis or transfer.**
>
> **Today, the most important problem in cancer treatment is how to resist metastasis. If the problem of cancer metastasis cannot be solved, cancer treatment cannot leap forward. Therefore, one of the goals of cancer treatment in the 21st century should be metastasis resistance.**

The results series of anti-cancer, anti-cancer metastasis research, scientific and technological innovation, scientific research

(7) Main features of the new concept of cancer treatment:

To control transfer or to control metastasis

XZ-C believes:

It is to control metastasis and to protect patient's immunity, not simply kill cancer cells.

Summary

a. How is it to control the metastasis or transfer?

Killing cancer cells in the human body should rely on two forces:

One is the external forces of surgery, radiotherapy, and chemotherapy;

the second is the internal strength of the patient's own immune function.

Drugs, surgery, and various treatment techniques are important for the treatment of patients, but *the body's own immunity is even more important.*

Many problems must be solved by the patient's own strength, because the body has a complete anti-cancer system.

Why is it?

It is because the main feature of the new concept of cancer treatment is to control metastasis and protect the patient's immunity, rather than simply killing cancer cells.

(8) New concept of cancer metastasis treatment

The target of anti-metastasis should be for cancer cells on the way to metastasis.

This book first published a new theoretical understanding internationally, that is, it was proposed a new concept of cancer anti-metastatic treatment:

There are three manifestations of cancer in the human body:

The first type is primary cancer;

The second type is metastatic cancer;

The third type is a group of cancer cells on the way to metastasis.

The target of anti-metastasis or the "target" of treatment should be targeted at the cancer cell population on the way to metastasis.

In fact, the key to anti-cancer metastasis is to encircle, block or interfere with the cancer cell population on the way to metastasis. Or the cancer cell group on the way of metastasis should be encircled, blocked or interfered.

The mode of the new treatment that cuts off the metastasis pathway is the key to fighting cancer metastasis.

According to the way of cancer cell metastasis, the model of the new anti-metastatic treatment is designed to destroy and block.

Why is it?

It is because the third manifestation is cancer cells, cancer cell populations and microcancer thrombus that are on the way to metastasis. Designing the model of the new anti-metastasis treatment aims at blocking the cancer cell population on the way to metastasis. This new theory proposed will conquer cancer metastasis and bring new hope.

(9) **New concept of cancer metastasis treatment**

The third form of cancer present or existing in the human body is the group of cancer cells on the way to metastasis

This book first discovered and proposed a new theory or new theoretical understanding in the world:

It is proposed that there are three existing forms or manifestations of cancer in the human body, and the third form of manifestation in the human body is the group of cancer cells that are on the way to metastasis.

The main manifestations of cancer in the human body, two different concepts of cancer treatment, there are two different understandings:

(1) XUZE's new concept of cancer treatment believes that there are three existing forms of cancer, and there are three manifestations of cancer in the human body:

The first existing form or manifestation: primary cancer;

The second existing form or manifestation: metastatic cancer;

Thethird existing or manifestation: cancer cells, cancer cell groups, and microcancer thrombi that are in the process of metastasis.

The goal or "target" of treatment is also for these three manifestations:

One is for the first manifestation-------primary cancer;

The second is for the second manifestation------metastatic cancer;

The third is for the third manifestation-----cancer cell populations on the way to metastasis.

This new concept believes that cancer exists three forms or is manifested in three forms in the human body, which is relatively complete and comprehensive. It clarifies the dynamic relationship, causality and subordination between the three, and is a complete new concept of cancer treatment. It fully explains the whole process of cancer development and how to control the whole process of cancer cell metastasis.

This new doctrine will bring the dawn of victory over cancer.

(2) The traditional concept of cancer therapy believes that there are two manifestations:

The first manifestation-----primary cancer;

The second manifestation-----metastatic cancer.

The traditional goals or "targets" of cancer therapy are for these two forms:

One is for the first manifestation----primary cancer;

The second is for the second manifestation-----metastatic cancer.

This traditional therapeutic concept has been used for more than one hundred years, and its treatment goals or "targets" are for these two manifestations-primary cancer or metastatic cancer. And it was to ignore the cancer cells on the way of metastasis.

As we all know, metastasis is the biological characteristics and biological behavior of malignant tumors.

The difference between benign and dangerous tumors and malignant tumors is that the former does not metastasize while the latter metastasizes. Anti-metastasis is the key to cancer treatment.

Without blocking the cancer cells in the process of metastasis, the metastasis of cancer cells cannot be controlled, and therefore, it is difficult to obtain the possibility of full cancer treatment.

(10) **New concept of cancer metastasis treatment**

"Two Points and One Line"

Summary

This book first proposes another new theory or new theoretical understanding in the world:

The "two points and one line" theory of the whole process of cancer development.

It is believed that in cancer treatment, only two points have been recognized and valued at home and abroad in the past and present, and the first line has been ignored.

In fact, cancer treatment should not only pay attention to two points, but also pay more attention to the one-line. Cutting off the one-line is just the key to fighting cancer metastasis.

What is two points and one line?

The two points are the starting point of metastasis, the primary cancer; and the end of metastasis, the metastatic cancer.

The one-line is a route between the primary cancer foci and the metastatic cancer foci where cancer cells travel a long distance to metastasize to distant organs. (Figure as the following)

Invasion and metastasis route

Primary cancer ⟶ B ⟶ Metastatic cancer

A   C

Schematic diagram for two-point and one-line of the whole process of cancer cell metastasis

Note:

A. Primary cancer, starting point of metastasis;
B. Route of invasion and transfer;
C. Metastatic cancer foci and end of metastasis.

Traditional cancer treatment often only pays attention to "two points", but ignores the "one line".

XU ZE's new concept of cancer treatment believes that it not only should pay attention to "two points", but also it should cut off the one line.

In summary, it can be seen that the new concept of XU ZE cancer treatment not only attaches importance to the surgical removal of primary and metastatic tumors, radiotherapy, and chemotherapy, but also pays more attention to the interception and killing of cancer cells on the way of metastasis.

This new theory, called "two points and one line", has the following important meanings:

It is to emphasize that anti-metastasis should not only pay attention to the "two points", but also pay more attention to the "first line".

Only by cutting off the cancer cells on the way of metastasis can the curative effect of cancer be improved.

(11) The "Three Steps" of Cancer Metastasis Treatment

Summary

How to resist metastasis?

The transfer steps should be understood to make the goal of treatment more specific.

This book summarizes the ***extremely complex, dynamic, continuous, multi-step, and multi-factor biological process*** of cancer cell metastasis, and puts forward the "eight-step" theory of cancer cell metastasis. In order to carry out scientific design, block each metastasis step, and defeat each step. Based on the "eight steps" and "three stages" discussing the molecular mechanism of cancer cell metastasis, the author designed and formulated prevention and treatment strategies for each stage, called anti-cancer metastasis therapy "Trilogy".

The first step in anti-cancer metastasis, the goal of prevention and treatment is to prevent cancer cells from entering the blood vessels to achieve the goal of "guarding against the enemy outside the country".

The second step of anti-cancer metastasis, the goal of prevention and treatment is to activate immune cells, protect the function of thymus tissue, enhance immunity, protect the marrow and produce blood, and encourage cancer cells floating in the vascular circulation to be captured, swallowed, and wiped out by immune cells.

The third step of anti-cancer metastasis, prevention and treatment goals: to improve local microenvironmental tissue immunity, make it difficult for cancer cells to implant, inhibit angiogenic factors, and inhibit the formation of new blood vessels.

Why is it?

The above-mentioned "three steps" of anti-cancer metastasis therapy *locates the space for the treatment of cancer metastasis in the blood circulation and the time in three different stages, with emphasis on enhancing the host's immunity and regulating the local microenvironment.*

The "trilogy" of anti-cancer metastasis therapy locates the space for the treatment of cancer metastasis in the blood circulation and the time in three different stages.

The focus is on enhancing host immunity, which can be summarized in Table and Figure as the following:

Table 1 "Trilogy" of anti-cancer metastasis treatment

Cancer metastasis stage	The route of metastais	Prevention countermeasures
Cancer cells invade the pre-circulatory stage, The first step of anti-metastatic	Separation of cancer cells from primary cancer Lower ECM Adhesion and de-adhesion movement Before entering the blood vessel	Anti-adhesion • Anti-degradation • Anti-exercise • Anti-matrix metalloproteinase • Keep cancer cells out of blood vessels
Cancer cells are transported in the blood circulation stage, The second step	Cancer cells and tiny tumor thrombi float in the blood circulation, it is undergone by phagocytosis and it is captured by immune cells, and the impact of blood shear force causes loss	• Enhance and activate various immune cells and immune factors in the circulation, enhance immune function, and become the main battlefield for annihilating cancer cells on the way to metastasis • Anti-adhesion • Anti-platelet aggregation • Anticancer thrombus

	Cancer cells escape the blood circulation. After the cancer cells escape the blood vessels, they anchor the "target" organs and anchor the "target" organs and tissues, and they will be implanted, and new blood vessels will be formed.	• Huang Lateng Ethyl Acetate Extract (TG) • Inhibit angiogenesis factor • Inhibit blood vessel formation • Increase immune regulation • Improve local microenvironmental tissue immunity

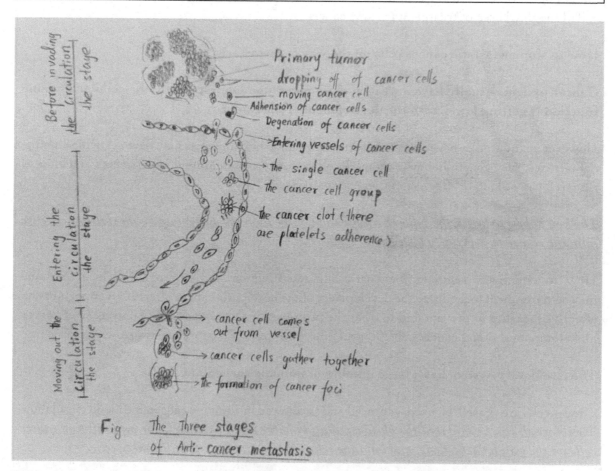

Primary tumor/Shed cancer cells/Adherence/Degraded ECM/
Cancer cells penetrate blood vessels/Pre-invasion cycle/Post-invasion stage/Single cancer cell/Cancer cell population/ Cancer thrombus (with platelet adhesion)/ Post-vascularization/Cancer cells penetrate blood vessels/Cancer cell aggregation/ Metastasis formation

Figure Three stages of anti-cancer metastasis

(12) **The new concept of treatment for cancer metastasis**

It is to open up the third field of treatment for anti-cancer metastasis

[Summary]

This book first proposes to open up the third field of human anti-cancer metastasis treatment in the world

What is the third field of therapy for anti-cancer metastasis?

It is the therapy that everything aims at the third existing form or manifestation of cancer in the human body, that is, it is the treatment of cancer cells in the process of metastasis, which can be called the third area of treatment for anti-cancer.

How to stop metastatic cancer cells on the way to metastasis?

Cancer patients usually have a weakened immune function, especially the cellular immune function is getting lower with the development of the tumor.

However, many studies have shown that although tumor-bearing hosts may have systemic immune deficiencies, they generally have normal T cell responses. Both animal experiments and clinical research can stimulate effective anti-cancer responses.

The key is how to break the tumor's suppression of the immune system and stimulate an effective immune response, especially based on T cells.

How to effectively regulate the host's immune function and improve the local immune microenvironment to facilitate the development of the host's anti-cancer effect is an important and effective measure to prevent and to treat the postoperative metastasis and recurrence of cancer and eliminate residual cancer cells. It is an important part of comprehensive cancer treatment.

The circulatory system has a large number of immune surveillance cells

Cancer cells are chased, blocked, captured and swallowed by immune cells in the blood circulation. Therefore, *it can be said that the blood circulation is the main battlefield for annihilating cancer cells on the way to metastasis, and immune cells are the vital force to kill cancer cells.*

The circulatory system has a large number of immune surveillance cells, which can kill and swallow cancer cells with heterogeneous antigens. Coupled with the impact and shear force of the bloodstream, it is difficult for a single swimming cancer cell to survive.

In order to escape the pursuit of immune cells, cancer cells are attached to the inner wall of blood vessels with platelets. The endothelial cells in the inner wall of the blood vessels make amoebic movement, pass through the capillaries and settle in new organs, gradually forming new metastases.

> The above-mentioned cancer cells in the metastasis process are actually the third manifestation in the human body, and we must find countermeasures. The third area of anti-cancer treatment is really necessary.

(13) Experimental screening of XZ-C immunomodulatory anti-cancer Chinese medicine

Summary

XZ-C immunomodulatory anti-cancer Chinese medicine is based on traditional Chinese herbal medicines in our country, and we have conducted experimental research on screening new anti-cancer and anti-metastatic drugs from Chinese medicines in our laboratory:

1. In vitro screening test:

The cancer cells were cultured in vitro to observe the direct damage of cell drugs to cancer cells.

2. The screening experiment of in vivo tumor suppression:

It was to create a cancer-bearing animal model, and carry out the anti-tumor rate of Chinese herbal medicine in cancer-bearing animals.

3. Experimental results:

Among the 200 Chinese herbal medicines screened out by animal experiments in our laboratory, 48 kinds of Chinese herbal medicines were screened out to have certain or even excellent inhibitory effects on cancer cells, with an inhibitory rate of 75-95% or more.

This group has been screened by animal experiments to eliminate 152 species without anticancer effects.

The main pharmacological effects of XZ-C immune regulation and anti-cancer Chinese medicine are "Thymus protection and increase immunity" and "bone marrow protection and blood production".

(14) Cancer treatment methods and drugs ----- A, B. C, D

A. One of the experimental screenings of XZ-C immunomodulatory anti-cancer Chinese medicine

Our laboratory has carried out the following experimental studies to screen new anti-cancer and anti-metastatic drugs from Chinese medicine:

(A) Use the method of in vitro culture of cancer cells to carry out the screening experiment of the anticancer rate of Chinese herbal medicine

In vitro screening test:

The cancer cells are cultured in vitro to observe the direct damage of the drugs to the cancer cells.

In the test tube screening test, put crude biological products (500ug/ml) into the test tubes for culturing cancer cells to observe whether they have inhibitory effects on cancer cells. We will conduct in vitro screening test one by one for 200 kinds of Chinese herbal medicines that traditional Chinese medicine was considered to have anti-cancer effects. They were cultured with normal fibroblasts under the same conditions to test the toxicity of the drug to such cells and then compare them.

(B) To create a tumor-bearing animal model and conduct an experimental screening study on the anti-cancer rate of Chinese herbal medicine in cancer-bearing animals.

Each batch of experiment uses 240 mice, divided into 8 groups, each group has 30 mice, the 7th group is the blank control group, the 8th group uses 5-FU or CTX as the control group, the whole group of mice is inoculated with EAC or siso or H22 cancer cell.

After 24 hours of inoculation, each rat was orally fed with crude crude drug powder, and fed with the selected traditional Chinese medicine for a long time to observe the survival period, toxicity and side effects, calculate the prolonged survival rate, and calculate the cancer suppression rate. In this way, we conducted 4 consecutive years of experimental research, and 3 years of experimental research on the pathogenesis, metastasis, and recurrence mechanisms of tumor-bearing mice, as well as experimental research to explore why tumors cause the death of the host. More than 1,000 model of tumor-bearing animals are used every year, nearly 6000 tumor-bearing animal models have been made in 4 years. After the death of each experimental mouse, pathological anatomy of the liver, spleen, lung, thymus, and kidney was performed, and more than 20,000 sections were performed to explore whether there may be micro-pathogens that may cause cancer. *Microcirculation microscope was used to observe the tumor microvascular establishment and microcirculation in 100 tumor-bearing mice.*

B. The second experimental screening of XZ-C immunomodulatory anti-cancer Chinese medicine

Through experimental research, we found that the traditional Chinese medicine TG has a significant effect in inhibiting tumor microvascular formation for the first time in China. It has been used in clinical anti-metastasis treatment for more than 80 patients, and the efficacy is being observed.

Experimental results

Among the 200 Chinese herbal medicines screened by animal experiments in our laboratory, 48 kinds of Chinese herbal medicines were screened to have certain or even excellent inhibitory effects on the proliferation of cancer cells, and the tumor inhibition rate was above 75-90%.

However, there are also some commonly used Chinese medicines that are generally considered to have anticancer effects. They have no anticancer effects after screening in vitro and in vivo tumor inhibition rates, or have little effect. This group has screened out 152 kinds of anticancer effects through animal experiments.

The 48 traditional Chinese medicines with good cancer suppression rate selected from this experiment were optimized and combined to repeat the cancer-bearing tumor suppression rate experiment.

__Finally, an anti-cancer Chinese medicine XU ZE China1-10 preparation (XZ-C1-10) with Chinese characteristics for immune regulation was developed.__

__XZ-C1 can significantly inhibit cancer cells, but does not affect normal cells; XZ-C4 can promote thymic hyperplasia and increase immunity; XZ-C8 can protect the blood of the marrow and protect the hematopoietic function of bone marrow.__

C. The third experimental screening of XZ-C immune regulation and anti-cancer Chinese medicine

Clinical validation

Clinical verification is carried out on the basis of successful animal experiments. That is, to establish an oncology specialist outpatient clinic and a combined anti-cancer, anti-metastasis, and recurrence scientific research team, **retain outpatient medical records, establish a regular follow-up observation system, and observe long-term effects.** From experimental research to clinical verification, new problems were discovered in the process of clinical verification, and then returned to the laboratory for basic research, and then applied the new experimental results to clinical verification. In this way, experiment one clinical, repeated experiment and repeated clinical, all experimental research must pass clinical verification, in a large number of patients, observation for 3-5 years, even 8-10 years of clinical observation,

According to circulatory medicine, there are long-term follow-up and evaluable data, and the evidence is clear that there is indeed a good long-term curative effect.

__The standard of curative effect is: the best survival quality and long survival period.__

XZ-C immunomodulatory anti-cancer Chinese medicine preparations have been verified by a large number of patients with advanced cancer, and have achieved significant effects.

XZ-C immune regulation and control Chinese medicine can improve the survival quality of patients with advanced cancer, enhance immunity, increase the body's anti-cancer ability, increase appetite, and significantly prolong survival.

D. The fourth experimental Screening of XZ-C Immunomodulation of anti-cancer Chinese Medicine

Clinical verification

1. Among the 4277 cases of advanced cancer patients who received XZ-C1-10 immunoregulatory Chinese medicine for more than 3 months of follow-up diagnosis, the medical records have detailed observation records of the efficacy, see the table below

Observation of the curative effect of 4277 cases to improve the quality of life of patients with advanced cancer

Improvement	spirit	Appetite	Strengthen	Weight gain	General conditions improve	Sleep better	Improvement activities Limited relief Self-care Walking activity As usual	Ability activity Return to work Doing light work
Number of cases	4071	3986	2450	479	2938	1005	1038	3220	479
(%)	95.2	93.2	57.3	11.2	68.7	23.5	24.3	75.3	11.2

2. For 84 cases of solid tumors and 56 cases of patients with metastatic supraclavicular lymphadenopathy, the XZ-C series and XZ-C3 anti-cancer light-hardening gel ointment were taken orally and XZ-C3 anti-cancer light-hardening knot ointment was applied to achieve better results. See the table below.

Changes of 84 cases of solid tumors and 56 cases of metastatic nodules after external application of XZ-C ointment

	Solid tumor mass				Swollen supraclavicular lymph nodes in the neck			
	Disappear	Reduce ½	Turn soft	no change	Disappear	Reduce ½	Turn soft	no change
Number of cases	12	28	32	12	12	22	14	8
(%)	14.2	33.3	38.0	14.2	21.4	39.2	25.0	14. 2
Total effective rate (%)	85.7				85.7			

3. Table of pain relief after oral administration of XZ-C drug and external application of XZ-C anticancer pain relief ointment in 298 patients

Clinical manifestations	Pain			
	Mild relief	Significantly reduced	disappear	invalid
Number of cases	52	139	93	14
(%)	17.3	46. 8	31.2	4.7
Total effective rate (%)	95.3%			

(15) Immunopharmacology of XZ-C immune regulation and control anticancer Chinese medication

Compared with western medicine immunopharmacology, Chinese medicine immunopharmacology has its own characteristics and advantages. After long-term clinical experience, Chinese medicine has accumulated a large number of prescriptions that can regulate the body's immune function, especially tonic Chinese medicines generally have the benefit of regulating immune vitality.

Traditional Chinese medicines, whether single-medicine or prescriptions, will have multiple active ingredients, unlike Western medicine (synthetic medicine) that has a single structure.

The role of traditional Chinese medicine is multifaceted. In addition to regulating immune function, it also has a certain effect on the overall functional system.

The main role of XZ-C Chinese medicine immunomodulator is to regulate cellular immunity (Cellular immunity) to regulate various immune cell-mediated immune responses, including cytokines or lymphokines.

The immune regulation function of Chinese medicine is also mainly used for stem cell immunity, such as thymus, gonads and lymphatic system, T, B cells and various cytokines.

Ancient Chinese medicine has the notion that righteous qi is not weak and evil qi is not invaded. It forms part of the theory of traditional Chinese medicine. Its essence is to maintain overall functional balance and enhance disease resistance. Its main function is to enhance the body's immune function. In fact, tonic drugs are based on immunopharmacology.

Immunopharmacology is an emerging edge subject, which serves as a bridge between pharmacology and immunology.

The traditional Chinese medicine of XZ-C immunomodulator has obvious immune promoting effect.

(16) **The adaptation scope for XZ-C1-10 immune regulation and control Chinese medicine anti-cancer metastasis and recurrence clinical application observation**

1. Various distant metastatic cancers:

Such as liver metastasis, lung metastasis, bone metastasis, brain metastasis, abdominal lymph node metastasis, mediastinal lymph node metastasis, cancerous pleural effusion, cancerous ascites, can come to the Wuchang Shuguang Oncology Specialty Clinic to apply XZ-C immunomodulation anti-metastasis therapy, anti-metastasis steps, intervention and blocking of cancer cells on the way of metastasis to prolong life.

2. After completing the course of various radiotherapy and chemotherapy, it should continue to come to the clinic to take XZ-C1-4 immunoregulatory Chinese medicine to consolidate the long-term effect and prevent recurrence.

3. In the course of radiotherapy and chemotherapy, if the reaction is severe and cannot be continued, they can come to the Shuguang Oncology Clinic and continue to use XZ-C immunomodulation therapy to prevent metastasis and recurrence.

4. For those who are elderly or infirm with other diseases who cannot undergo radiotherapy or chemotherapy, they can come to the Shuguang Oncology

Specialty Clinic to use XZ-C immune regulation for anti-metastasis and recurrence treatment.

5. For those who cannot be removed by surgical exploration, they can come to Shuguang Cancer Specialist Clinic XZ-C immunoregulatory treatment.

6. After palliative surgery, they can come to Shuguang Oncology Specialty Clinic for XZ-C immunomodulation anti-metastasis therapy.

7. After radical resection of various cancers, they can continue to take XZ-C immunomodulatory anti-cancer Chinese medicine to prevent metastasis and recurrence in the outpatient clinic to improve the long-term efficacy.

Secret level: Grade A

(17) Research on XZ-C immune regulation and control anti-cancer Chinese medication

Table of Contents

1. Overview

2. The experimental research and clinical verification work that has been carried out

3. The immune pharmacology of XZ-C immune regulation and control Chinese medicine

4. The research of XZ-C immunomodulatory anti-cancer Chinese medicine pharmacodynamics

5. The research of XZ-C4 anti-cancer traditional Chinese medicine induced cytokine

6. The research of XZ-C immune regulation and control anti-cancer traditional Chinese medicine toxicology

7. About the active ingredients of XZ-C immune regulation anti-cancer Chinese medicine

8. XZ-C prescription principles

9. About the immune function of XZ-C drug immune regulation and anti-cancer Chinese medicine at the molecular level

10. About the anti-tumor components of XZ-C drug immune regulation and control anti-cancer Chinese medicine: structural formula, location, anti-tumor effect

11. The source background and completion process of the subject (tortuous process)

12. How can I get out of the boudoir?

(18)

a. **The cases list of XZ-C immune regulation and control anti-cancer Chinese medicine treatment of cancer**

Table of Contents

7. List of some cases of **colorectal cancer** treated with XZ-C immune regulation anti-cancer Chinese medicine
(Case 482------Case 649)

8. List of some cases of XZ-C immunoregulatory anti-cancer Chinese medicine for treatment of **cholangiocarcinoma**
(Case 650-----Case 679)

b. **Some typical cases of XZ-C immunoregulatory anti-cancer Chinese medicine for treatment of malignant tumors**

Table of Contents

1. Treatment of some typical cases of **liver cancer**

2. Some typical cases of postoperative adjuvant treatment of **pancreatic** cancer

3. Some typical cases of adjuvant treatment after **gastric** cancer

4. Some typical cases of postoperative adjuvant treatment of **lung cancer**

5. Some typical cases of postoperative adjuvant treatment of **esophageal cancer**

6. Some typical cases of adjuvant treatment after **breast cancer surgery**

7. Some typical cases of postoperative adjuvant treatment of colorectal cancer

8. Some typical cases of adjuvant treatment after gallbladder cancer

9. Some typical cases of adjuvant treatment after renal cancer and bladder cancer

10. Some typical cases of postoperative adjuvant treatment such as thyroid cancer and retroperitoneal tumors

11. Some typical cases of non-Hodgkin's lymphoma treatment

12. A typical case of chemotherapy + XZ-C Chinese medicine in the treatment of acute **lymphoblastic leukemia**

13. Some typical cases of ovarian cancer and cervical cancer treatment

Strive to take the innovative path of anti-cancer metastasis with Chinese characteristics!

Take the path of Chinese medicine modernization, promote the integration of Chinese and Western medicine at the molecular level, and integrate with international medicine modernization!

(19) The theoretical system of XZ-C treatment has been formed

The book "New Concepts and New Methods of Cancer Treatment" published that Professor Xu Ze spent 60 years on his own and worked hard to complete the basic and clinical research of the National Science and Technology Commission's "Eighth Five-Year Plan" research topics.

Nearly a hundred scientific research papers summarized by a series of scientific research results were published in the form of a new book.

This book has formed the theoretical system of XZ-C cancer treatment, which is the theoretical basis and experimental basis for cancer treatment. It has been undergoing clinical application observation and verification.

XZ-C laboratory animal experiment found:

1. It can create a cancer animal model after the removal of the thymus

2. As the cancer progresses, the thymus gland gradually shrinks

---

↓

It was found the disease cause or etiology:

thymus atrophy and weakened immune function

↓

It was put forward the theory of treatment based on:

XZ-C immune regulation and control

Protection of Thymus and increase Immune function

↓

The exclusively developed products:

XZ-C immune regulation preparation 1-10

↓

Clinical verification:

Over the past 18 years, outpatient observation and follow-up of more than 12,000 patients with advanced cancer have been able to improve the quality of life, prolong the survival period, and have satisfactory results

XZ-C Theoretical System of Cancer Treatment

(XZ-C) (XU ZE-China)

(20) **This book proposed the new concept of XZ-C cancer therapy, which was analyzed and compared with traditional therapy. This analysis is showed as the following Table:**

	XZ-C new concept of cancer therapy	Traditional Chemotherapy Cancer Therapy
Theoretical basis	The new concept believes: Healing should be through regulation rather than killing	The traditional concept is that: the goal of treatment must be to kill cancer cells
Etiology, pathogenesis	Thymus atrophy Immune function is weak	N

The theoretical basis and experimental basis of treatment	Immune regulation and control; Protection of Thymus and increase immune function	Not yet
Treatment principles	Establish a comprehensive treatment view	Single target to kill cancer cells, one-sided treatment view
Treatment mode	Full treatment: surgery + biological immune regulation Short-term treatment: radiotherapy, chemotherapy Not long range Not excessive	Radiotherapy + chemotherapy Chemical + radiotherapy Or simultaneous radiotherapy and chemotherapy
medicine	XZ-C immune regulation 1+10 modernization of traditional Chinese medicine, molecular level combination of Chinese and Western	Cytotoxic drugs (killing both cancer cells and normal proliferating cells)
Complications, side effects	No	Toxic side effects, Some have serious side effects, Some even weakened immune function, Radiotherapy damage is permanent.
Curative effect	Improve quality of life and prolong survival	Relief for a few months and may relapse and progress
Medical cost	Greatly reduced medical expenses	The cost of medicine is large, nearly 100 billion yuan per year in my country
prospect	Walked out the new path to overcome cancer	The effect is 5%, still lingering

(21) **What are the reforms in the book? What are the innovations?**

The third monograph "New Concepts and New Methods of Cancer Treatment" is an innovative concept and content, which has both experimental research basis and clinically verified "New Concepts of Cancer Therapy".

1). **The following are the reforms and innovations of traditional therapy proposed by XZ-C internationally or nationally:**

(1) Now the whole world is a single cancer cell killing, which is a one-sided treatment. **XU proposes to reform into a comprehensive treatment.**

(2) Now that the whole world is dominated by radiotherapy and chemotherapy, **the XU proposal should be reformed into surgery + immune regulation as the main**, and radiotherapy and chemotherapy as supplementary.

(3) The whole world is now systemic intravenous chemotherapy for solid tumors. XU proposes to reform *into target organ intravascular* chemotherapy.

(4) Currently chemotherapeutics are not selective, and should be researched and innovated as *selective intelligent anticancer drugs, XZ-C1-4 is selective.*

(5) *There is no susceptibility to chemotherapy at present, XU suggests that a susceptibility test should be done (to avoid blindness).*

(6) At present, all tumor specimens have not been cultured for cancer cells. XU suggested that **all tumor specimens should be cultured for cancer cells (individualized and selective).**

(7) The design of radical resection should be further studied and improved. XU pointed out that the current radical resection is flawed. Several metastasis approaches only pay attention to the solution of lymphatic metastasis, *as well as blood circulation and implantation. Technology, pay attention to tumor-free technology to prevent the blood spread of cancer cells during surgery.*

(8) Now postoperative chemotherapy is mostly carried out in the chemotherapy department. The chemotherapy doctors and nurses do not understand the conditions seen during the operation.

XU proposes that postoperative chemotherapy should be postoperative adjuvant chemotherapy or perioperative adjuvant chemotherapy should be reformed as **the surgeon and Surgical nurses do it, because the surgeon can grasp the whole process of treatment after the drug pump administration, observation, and follow-up.**

(9) For half a century, traditional therapies believe that radiotherapy and chemotherapy are based on killing cancer cells. *This book proposes that the cure should be through regulation and control rather than killing.*

The achievement series of anti-cancer, anti-cancer metastasis research, scientific and technological innovation, scientific research

2). **The following arguments in this book are the first to be put forward in the world, all of which are original papers, leading the world:**

(1) It is the first in the world to propose: **Thymus atrophy and low immune function are the causes and pathogenesis of cancer.**

This is the internationally leading achievement of independent intellectual property rights. After a novelty search, this is the first time that it has been proposed in the world.

(2) The first in the world to propose: XZ-C immunomodulation therapy *--- Thymus protection and immune function increase, which is the theoretical basis and experimental basis for cancer treatment.*

(3) The first international initiative: the goal or target of cancer treatment must be aimed at *both the tumor and the host, and a comprehensive treatment view must be established.* The one-sided treatment view of simply killing cancer cells should be overcome.

(4) The first international initiative: the multi-disciplinary organic integration model is mainly *long-term treatment: surgery + biological treatment ten immunotherapy. Short-term treatment is supplemented: radiotherapy and chemotherapy, not long-term, not excessive.*

(5) The first in the world to point out: **the problems and disadvantages of systemic intravenous chemotherapy for solid tumors, questioning and four comments.**

(6) The first international proposal: It is recommended that systemic intravenous chemotherapy for solid abdominal tumors should be reformed *into target organ intravascular chemotherapy*.

(7) It is the first in the world to propose: *There are three main manifestations of cancer in the human body, and the third form is cancer cells that are in the process of metastasis.*

(8) The first in the world to propose: the *"two points and one line" theory of the whole process of cancer development. Cancer treatment should pay attention to two points and cut the line.*

(9) The first in the world to propose: **a three-step anti-cancer metastasis treatment, and three major strategies for anti-cancer metastasis treatment.**

(10)   The first international proposal*: it is to open up the third area of anti-cancer treatment.*

3). **The following arguments in this book are first proposed nationwide:**

(1) Animal experiments in our experimental surgery laboratory explore the cause, pathogenesis, and pathophysiology of cancer. Since 1985, the results and scale have been the first in the country.

(2) Excision of the thymus to create animal models, and use cancer-bearing animal models to conduct in vitro and in vivo anti-tumor experiments with traditional Chinese medicines. 48 Chinese medicines of XZ-C have been screened out from 200 kinds of Chinese medicines through in vivo experiments in tumor-bearing animal models, which should be domestically advanced and internationally advanced.

(3) The medical records of specialist outpatient clinics have been kept for 18 years, with more than 12,000 cases, follow-up, long-term follow-up, and establishment of cancer clinic medical records database.

(4) The exclusively developed XZ-C immunomodulatory Chinese medicine 1-10 has been clinically verified for 18 years, and has achieved good results after long-term observation and follow-up.

4). XZ-C proposes the following reform and development proposals for traditional therapy:

In the last two centuries, there have been two leaps in the treatment of malignant tumors

↓

The first time was when Halsted proposed the concept of radical tumor resection in 1890

↓

The second time was Fish integrated chemotherapy into radical surgery in the 1970s
(Adjuvant chemotherapy or neoadjuvant chemotherapy)

↓

Since then, the treatment of malignant tumors has been stagnant,
and the death of malignant bell tumor is still the first

Radical mastectomy	Chemotherapy is integrated into radical mastectomy (Adjuvant chemotherapy or neoadjuvant chemotherapy)
↓	↓
Extended radical mastectomy Super radical mastectomy	Radiation and chemotherapy target to kill cancer cells, Kill proliferating cells and immune cells at the same time
↓	↓
Modified radical mastectomy	It fails to improve the curative effect, and toxic side effects occur, which reduces immunity

Professor Xu Ze puts forward the following 4 suggestions for reform and development:	Professor Xu Ze proposed the following 6 reform and development proposals:
1. It is proposed that the design of radical surgery needs further research and improvement.	*1. Point out that the cure should be through regulation, not just killing*
2. It was proposed that tumor-free technology in tumor surgery is extremely important.	*2. A comprehensive treatment should be established for both the host and cancer cells*
3. During the operation, it should prevent the blood spreading of cancer cells.	*3. Point out that chemotherapy needs to be further researched and improved*
4. During the operation, it should prevent shedding cancer cells to cause cancer planting.	*4. Questions the administration route of systemic intravenous chemotherapy for solid tumors*
	5. Advocate the reform of systemic intravenous chemotherapy for solid tumors into target organ intravascular chemotherapy
	6. Advocate the reform of adjuvant chemotherapy after cancer surgery to omental vein catheter pump chemotherapy.

5). The following first published original papers are published in this book:

1). One of the etiology and pathogenesis of cancer may be thymic atrophy and weakened immune function. (chapter 2)

2). The theoretical basis and experimental basis of the therapeutic principles of XZ-C immune regulation and control therapy for Thymus protection and immune function promotion (Chapter 3).

3). Cancer treatment targets must be aimed at both the tumor and the host at the same time to establish a comprehensive treatment view (Chapter 5).

4). It is to propose a comprehensive treatment plan (Chapter 6).

The whole course treatment: mainly surgery + biological treatment, immunomodulation treatment

The short-term treatment: mainly radiotherapy and chemotherapy, not excessive

5). The analysis and questioning of the administration route of systemic intravenous chemotherapy for solid tumors (Chapter 11).

6). The proposal that systemic intravenous chemotherapy for solid tumors should be reformed into target organ intravascular chemotherapy (Chapter 12).

These six original papers proposed a series of reforms and innovations on traditional chemotherapy and chemotherapy.

7). Resection of the thymus to create animal models, use cancer-bearing animal models for in vitro and in vivo Chinese medicine anti-tumor experiments, screen out 48 Chinese medicines of XZ-C from 200 kinds of Chinese medicines through in vivo experiments on tumor-bearing animal models, and develop XZ-C1-10 Immune regulation anti-cancer Chinese medicine preparation.

8). XZ-C immune regulation anti-cancer Chinese medicine research overview, experimental research and clinical efficacy observation (Chapter 26 and Chapter 27).

9). Strategic thinking and suggestions for conquering cancer.

The above nine original scientific research papers may enable cancer treatment to embark on a new path to overcome cancer and move towards a new era of immune regulation and targeted therapy. This is not the end of subject research, but the beginning of a new path to translational medicine through the development of translational medicine.

Translational medicine has developed rapidly internationally in recent years. This new medical research model advocates patient-centeredness, discovering questions and asking questions from clinical work, conducting in-depth basic research, and then quickly turning the results of basic research into clinical applications to improve the overall level of medical care and ultimately benefit patients. The XZ-C series of scientific research results are fully in line with this new medical research model.

The focus of translational medicine research in my country, the modernization and internationalization of Chinese medicine and traditional Chinese medicine is one of the key contents of translational medicine research in my country.

It has been more than 15 years since the publication of this monograph and new book, we will start to organize the transformation and development of XZ-C scientific research results

2

The ideological understanding and scientific research thinking of our scientific research journey

Summary

Our years of thinking and understanding of the scientific journey of cancer research work and scientific research thinking can be divided into three stages. Introduction:

(1) **The first stage 1985-1999**

- From the results of the follow-up, the problem is found-the problem is raised-the research problem;
- From reviewing, analyzing, reflecting, and discovering the current problems of traditional cancer therapy, further research and improvement are needed;
- Recognizing that there are problems, you should change your thinking and concepts;
- Summarized the data, compiled, compiled, and published the first monograph "New Understanding and New Model of Cancer Treatment" published in January 2001 by Hubei Science and Technology Press.

(2) **The second stage after 2001-**

- Position the target of research and cancer treatment against metastasis, and point out that the key to cancer treatment is anti-metastasis;
- A series of anti-cancer metastasis and recurrence experimental research and clinical basic and clinical verification research have been carried out, and it has been upgraded to theoretical innovation, and new ideas and new methods for anti-metastasis have been proposed;

- Summarized the data, compiled, compiled, and published the second monograph "New Concepts and New Methods for Cancer Metastasis Treatment", published by People's Military Medical Publishing House in January 2006, and published by Xinhua Bookstore. In April 2007, it was awarded the General Publishing House of the People's Republic of China. "Three Hundreds" Original Book Award issued by the Ministry of Education.

(3) The third phase after 2006-

- Conduct research on the prevention and treatment of the entire process of cancer occurrence and development with the research objectives and focus;
- Tightly integrate clinical practice, and propose reforms and innovations, scientific research and development in response to the current problems and drawbacks of traditional clinical therapies;
- Recognizing that the strategy of cancer prevention and treatment must move forward, the way out for cancer treatment is in the "three mornings", and the way out for anti-cancer is prevention,
- It has been engaged in oncology surgery for 55 years. There are more and more patients, the incidence of cancer is also rising, and the mortality rate remains high. It was deeply realized that cancer should not only pay attention to treatment, but also pay attention to prevention, in order to stop at the source. It has conducted a series of related research, summarized materials, sorted out, compiled, and published the third monograph "New Concepts and New Methods of Cancer Treatment".

Science-is the endless frontier

Our scientific research work has always followed the scientific development concept, based on known science, facing the future of medicine, and looking forward. After 28 years of long-term hard work, we are facing the frontier of science and striving for innovation and progress. We deeply understand:

- To conquer cancer, we must come from the clinic, go through experimental research, and go to the clinic to solve the actual problems of patients;
- We must seek truth from facts, speak with facts and data; we must constantly surpass ourselves and advance ourselves;
- In scientific research, we should resolve ideological constraints, get rid of traditional old concepts, and base ourselves on independent innovation and original innovation;

- Our 20-year scientific research route is to discover problems→propose problems→research problems→solve problems or explain problems. The road is like this, step by step, and arduous journey. Under the guidance of the scientific development concept, we hope to create a path with China Features, an innovative path of anti-cancer and anti-metastasis with independent intellectual property rights.

- Our medical oncology research model is patient-centered, discovering and asking questions from clinical work, conducting in-depth basic research on animal experiments, and then turning the results of basic research into clinical applications to improve the overall level of medical care and ultimately benefit patients.

- Experimental surgery is extremely important in the development of medicine. It is a key to open the forbidden area of medicine. The prevention and treatment methods of many diseases have been applied in clinical practice and promote the development of medical undertakings after many animal experiments and studies have achieved stable results.

3

Experimental and Clinical Observation of XZ-C Immunomodulation Anti-cancer Chinese Medicine in Treating Malignant Tumor

In order to find anti-cancer Chinese medicines that have anti-cancer curative effects without toxic and side effects to the body, our Institute of Surgical Oncology,

The 200 kinds of Chinese herbal medicines with anti-cancer effects recorded in Chinese medicine books were screened one by one for anti-tumor effects of solid tumors in tumor-bearing animal models.

After a long-term batch of in vivo tumor suppression animal experiments, 48 kinds of Chinese herbal medicines that have a good tumor suppression rate and prolong survival, protect immune organs and significantly improve immune function have been screened out.

According to clinical case differentiation and treatment principles of strengthening the body and removing the evil, softening and dispelling the masses, and anti-cancer promotion and immunity, the selected anti-cancer drugs are combined into two compounds XZ-C1 and XZ-C4 that have better anti-cancer effects than each single agent.

The initial screening was a cancer-suppressing animal experiment for each single herbal medicine. Now we are going further to conduct further experimental research on the anti-tumor effect of the two groups of compound prescriptions on solid tumors in tumor-bearing mice.

1). Animal Experimental Research

1)). Materials and methods

(1) Laboratory animals

There are 260 pure Kunming mice, half male and half, weighing 21 ± 2g, 8-10 weeks old.

(2) Tumor strain and inoculation:

Liver cancer H22 tumor line, take the fresh tumor body of the tumor-bearing mouse to make a single cell suspension. After the cancer cells are stained and counted (1X106/ml), 0.2 ml of normal saline for the cancer cells is placed under the right anterior axillary skin of each mouse Vaccination.

(3) Drug and experiment group:

The traditional Chinese medicine XZ-C1 and XZ-C4 are both developed and developed by the Anti-Cancer Collaborative Group. The former is a mixture, the latter is a powder (infusion), and the chemotherapy control drug used in the chemotherapy group is cyclophosphamide (CTX).

Experiment grouping:

The H22 cancer cell transplanted animals were randomly divided into four groups:

① The mice in the traditional Chinese medicine XZ-C1 group (90 mice) were intragastrically administered once a day 24 hours after cancer cell transplantation, each time 0.8ml/mouse, which is equivalent to 1.4mg crude drug.

② The traditional Chinese medicine XZ-C4 group (90 animals), the dosage and the method of gavage are the same as above.

③ The chemotherapy group (50 animals) started on the next day after cancer cell transplantation and was given CTX 50 mg/kg body weight every other day.

④ Control group (30 rats), starting from the next day after cancer cell transplantation, 0.8ml of normal saline per day

(4) Observation index:

The body weight of the mice was measured every 3 days, the diameter of the tumor was measured with a vernier caliper, the immune function was measured, and the blood picture was measured.

Half of each group is group A. For the tumor-bearing experiment, the mice are executed in batches and the tumors are separated and the tumor weight is calculated to calculate the tumor inhibition rate. The tumor was made pathological section, and a few specimens were observed for ultrastructure.

Half of each group is group B, tumor-bearing experimental mice, long-term infusion, until their own death, and then separate the tumor mass to calculate the long-term tumor inhibition rate and life extension rate.

2)). Experimental results

(1) The anti-tumor effect of XZ-C Chinese medicine on H22 mice bearing liver cancer:

The tumor inhibition rate of XZ-C1 was 40% in the second week, 45% in the fourth week, and 58% in the sixth week.

The tumor inhibition rate of XZ-C4 was 55% in the second week, 68% in the fourth week, and 70% in the sixth week. (P<0.01)

In the second week of CTX medication, the tumor inhibition rate was 45%. The tumor inhibition rate was 45% at the 4th week, and 49% at the 6th week (Figure 1, Figure 2).

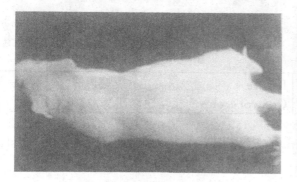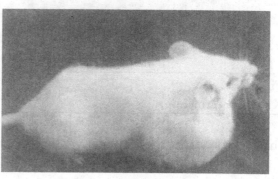

| Figure 1 XZ-C1, XZ-C4 treatment group 30 days after inoculation of liver cancer H22 | Figure 2 Control group 30 days after inoculation of liver cancer H22 |

(2) The effect of XZ-C Chinese medicine on the survival time of H22 mice bearing liver cancer XZ-C1, XZ-C4, and the average survival days of the CTX group were higher than those of the normal saline control group (P<0.01):

XZ-C Chinese medicine has the effect of prolonging survival period significantly.

Compared with the control group, the XZ-C1 life extension rate was 85%, the XZ-C4 group life extension rate was 200%, and the CTX group life extension rate was 9.8%.

Both XZ-C1 and CTX groups in group B died within 75 days.

In XZ-C4 group, 6 cancer-bearing mice were still alive after 7 months.

(3) XZ-C1 and XZ-C4 both increase immune function. XZ-C4 can significantly increase immune function, increase white blood cells and red blood cells, and has no effect on liver and kidney function, and no damage to liver and kidney slices.

CTX reduces white blood cells and reduces immune function. Kidney slices have kidney damage. The thymus in the control group was significantly atrophy (Figure 4).

The thymus in the XZ-C1 and XZ-C4 treatment groups did not shrink and was slightly enlarged (Figure 3)

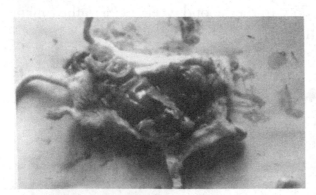 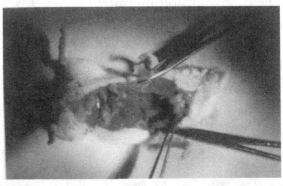

Figure 3 XZ-C4 treatment group	Figure 4 Control group

Thirty days after inoculation with liver cancer H22, the thymus glands are obviously enlarged

The thymus gland was significantly atrophy 30 days after inoculation with liver cancer H22

Pathological section of control thymus:

Thymus cortex is atrophy, cells are sparse, and blood vessels are congested (Figure). The XZ-C4 treatment group thymus pathology section showed thickening of the thymic cortex, dense lymphocytes, increased heptadermal reticulocytes, and increased thymic corpuscles (Figure 6).

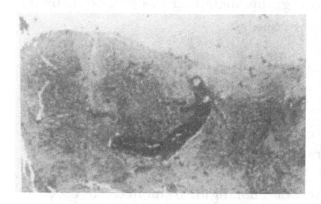

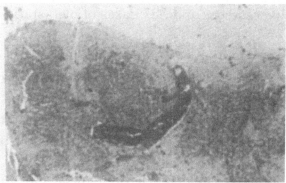

Figure 5	Figure 6
Pathological section of thymus in tumor-bearing control group HEX100	Thymus in XZ-C4 treatment group HEx100 Thymus cortex medulla is thickened and lymphocytes are highly dense
Cortical atrophy Lymphocytes are significantly reduced, a lymphocyte empty zone is formed in the cortex, and intravascular congestion	

2). Clinical application observation

1)). Clinical data

(1) In the Hubei Group of the National Collaborative Group of Integrated Chinese and Western Medicine Anti-cancer Research, the Anti-cancer Metastasis and Recurrence Research Laboratory, and the Shuguang Oncology Specialist Outpatient Department, from 1994 to November 2002, **XZ-C immunomodulatory anti-cancer Chinese medicine combined with Chinese and Western medicine was used to treat 4698 cases of stage III, IV or metastasis or recurrence, including 3051 males and 1647 females.**

The youngest is 11 years old, the oldest is 86 years old, and the age at high incidence is 40-59 years old.

All patients in the whole group are middle and advanced stage patients above stage III.

There were 1021 cases of liver cancer in this group, including 594 cases of primary liver cancer and 327 cases of metastatic liver cancer;

752 cases of lung cancer, including 699 cases of primary lung cancer and 53 cases of metastatic lung cancer; 668 cases of gastric cancer,

624 cases of esophagus and cardia cancer, 328 cases of rectal and anal canal cancer, 442 cases of colon cancer, 368 cases of breast cancer,

74 cases of pancreatic cancer, 30 cases of cholangiocarcinoma, 43 cases of retroperitoneal tumors, 38 cases of ovarian cancer, 9 cases of cervical cancer, 11 cases of brain tumors,34 cases of thyroid cancer,

38 cases of nasopharyngeal carcinoma, 9 cases of melanoma,

27 cases of kidney cancer, 48 cases of bladder cancer,

13 cases of leukemia, 47 cases of supraclavicular lymph node metastasis, 35 cases of various sarcomas, 39 cases of other malignant tumors.

   (2) Drugs and methods of administration:

The treatment is to strengthen the body and eliminate the evil, soften the firmness and dispel lumps, and tonic the qi and blood.

XZ-Cl is a mixture, 150ml per day, XZ-C4 is a powder (granule), 10g per day, according to the syndrome differentiation, solid tumors or metastatic tumors, both oral anticancer and external anticancer ointment.

For those with pain, apply topical anticancer pain relief cream.

For jaundice and ascites, use Tuihuangtang or Xiaoshuitang.

(3) Efficacy evaluation:

__Not only pay attention to short-term efficacy and imaging indicators, but also pay more attention to long-term efficacy, survival, quality of life and immune indicators.__

Pay attention to the change of subjective symptoms during the medication. It is effective if the subjective symptoms improve and last for more than 1 month, otherwise it is invalid. The improvement of the quality of life (Kafler score) also needs to continue for 1 month to be effective, otherwise it is invalid.

The evaluation criteria for the efficacy of solid tumor masses are divided into 4 levels according to the changes in tumor size:

Grade I: The mass disappeared;

Level II: Lump reduction class;

Class Ill: The lump becomes soft;

Grade IV: No change or enlargement of the mass.

2)). Treatment results

(1) *__It improved symptoms, improved quality of life, and prolonged survival:__*

Among the 4277 patients with intermediate and advanced cancer who took XZ-C immunoregulatory Chinese medicine for more than 3 months of follow-up visits, the medical records have detailed curative effect observation records, see Table 1; the quality of life of the patients has been improved, see Table 2.

Bin Wu and Lily Xu

Table 1. General Data of Recurrent and Metastasis of 4277 Cases

		Liver cancer	Lung cancer	Stomach cancer	Esophagus Cardia Cancer	Rectal anal cancer	Colon cancer	Breast cancer	Pancreatic cancer
Number of cases		1021	752	668	624	328	442	368	74
Male: female		4:1	44:1	2.25:1	3.1:1	1:1	2.1:1	All women	32:1
Cancer foci	Primary	694 (68.8%)	699 (93.9%)						
	Metastasis	327 (31.2%)	53 (6.1%)						
Common places of transfers in this group		Lung Metastasis (2%) From Stomach (27.2%) From the esophagus Cardia Bone	Supraclavicular lymph node metastasis (11.6%) Brain metastasis (3.1%) Bone	Metastatic liver (23.8%) Lung metastasis (3%) Peritoneal metastasis	Supraclavicular metastasis (13.1%) Liver metastasis (8.3%)	Recurrence rate (14.8%) Metastatic Liver (7.0%)	Metastatic liver (16.0%) Peritoneal Metastasis (6.0%)	Supraclavicular lymph node metastasis (175%) Axillary lymph node metastasis (15.0%) Bone metastasis (5.0%)	Metastatic liver (11.7%) etroperitoneal metastasis (39.1%)

Age	Cancer (19.5%) From the rectum (31.2%)	metastasis (4.6%)	(29.1%) Supraclavicular metastasis (6.1%)					
Peak age (years old) (%)	30-39 (76.2)	50-69 (71.6)	40-49 (73.4)	40-69 (80.4)	40-49 (75.2)	30-69 (88.0)	40-59 (55.9)	40-59 (70.0)
The Youngest (years old)	11	20	17	30	27	27	29	34
The oldest (years old)	86	80	77	77	78	76	80	68

Table 2 Observation of curative effect of 4277 cases to comprehensively improve the quality of life of advanced cancer patients

Aspects of Improvement	spirit	Appetite	Body Strengthen	General conditions	Weight gain	Sleep	Improve mobility, alleviate activity limitation	Take care of your own life and walk as usual	Return to work Doing light work
Number of improvement cases	4071	3986	2450	479	2938	1005	1038	3220	479
%	95.2	93.2	57.3	11.2	68.7	23.5	24.3	75.3	11.2

The patients in this group are all in the middle and advanced stages. They all have different degrees of symptom improvement after taking the medicine, with an effective rate of 93.2%. In terms of improving the quality of life (according to the Karnofsky score), the average score is 50 points before the medication and 80 points after the medication.

All patients in this group have metastasis and dysfunction of different organelle tubes above stage III. According to previous statistics, the median survival time of such patients is about 6 months.

The longest cases in this group have reached 28 years, and the average survival time of the remaining cases is more than 1 year.

1 case of primary liver cancer in the left lobe of the liver, recurred in the right liver after resection, and has been treated with XZ-C alone for 28 years;

Another case of liver cancer has been taking XZ-C for 20 and a half years;

In 2 cases of liver cancer, there were multiple cancers in the liver. After taking XZ-C for half a year, the cancers completely disappeared after 2 CT reexaminations, and they have been stable for half a year.

One case of double kidney cancer had extensive metastasis to the abdominal cavity after one side was excised. After taking XZ-C medicine, he has completely returned to work.

Three cases of lung cancer could not be cut through open chest examination, and they had been taking XZ-C medicine for three and a half years.

Two cases of remnant gastric cancer have been taking XZ-C medicine for 8 years.

3 cases of rectal cancer recurrence took XZ-C medicine for 3 years.

One case of breast cancer metastasized to liver and ribs has been taking medicine for 8 years.

One case of renal cancer recurred with bladder cancer after surgery, and the drug XZ-C disappeared for 9 and a half years.

__None of the above cases can be operated on, nor can they be treated with radiotherapy or chemotherapy. They are only treated with XZ-C drugs and not treated with other drugs.__

__So far, I still come to the clinic every month for review and medicine. After long-term medication, the condition is controlled in a stable state, so that the body and the tumor are in a balanced state for a long time, and a better survival with the tumor is obtained, the patient's symptoms are improved, the quality of life is improved, and the survival period is prolonged.__

(2) For 84 cases of solid masses and 56 cases of patients with metastatic supraclavicular lymphadenopathy, the XZ-C series which were taken orally and external application of XZ-C3 anti-cancer softening knot ointment have achieved good results. See Table 3.

	Solid mass	Swollen supraclavicular lymph nodes in the neck
	Disappear Reduce ½ Turn soft No change	Disappear Reduce 1/2 Turn soft No change
Number of cases	12 28 32 12	12 22 14 8

%	14.2 33.3 38.0 142		21.4 39.2 25.0 14.2
Total effective rate (%)	85.7		85.7

Table 3 Changes of 84 cases of solid masses and 56 cases of
metastatic nodules after external application of XZ-C ointment

(3) 298 cases of cancer pain patients took XZ-C medicine internally and applied XZ-C anticancer pain relief ointment to obtain significant analgesic effects. See Table 4.

Table 4 Pain relief after oral administration of XZ-C medicine and external application of XZ-C anticancer pain relief ointment in 298 patients

Clinical manifestations	Pain			
	Mild relief	Significantly reduced	Disappear	Invalid
Number of cases	52	139	93	14
(%)	17.3	46.8	31.2	4.7
Total effective rate (%)		95.3		

3). XZ-C immune regulation and control anti-cancer Chinese medicine experiment and clinical efficacy

1). XZ-C1-4 anti-cancer traditional Chinese medicine has anti-tumor effect on H22 tumor-bearing mice.

It was found that H22 tumor-bearing mice were treated for 2 weeks, 4 weeks, and 6 weeks after observation. The tumor inhibition rate increased with the prolonged medication time. The tumor inhibition rate of XZ-C4 was as high as 70% at the 6th week.

After two subsequent repeated tests, the results were stable, indicating that the anti-tumor effect of traditional Chinese medicine was slowly and gradually increased, that is, the anti-tumor effect was positively correlated with the cumulative dose of traditional Chinese medicine.

The effect of XZ-C1 and XZ-C4 anti-cancer Chinese medicine on the survival time of H22 tumor-bearing mice:

Experimental results prove that XZ-C1, XZC4 anti-cancer Chinese medicine can significantly prolong the survival time of tumor-bearing mice, especially XZ-C4, which significantly prolongs its survival time by more than 200%. Not only that, XZ-C4 can also significantly improve the immune function of the body It protects the immune organs, protects the bone marrow, and reduces the side effects of chemotherapy and radiotherapy drugs. It has been fed to mice for up to 12 months without any side effects.

The above experimental research provides a beneficial basis for clinical application.

2). Clinical efficacy

On the basis of experimental research, it has been applied to various types of clinical cancers since 1994, mostly in patients with stage III and IV or above, namely:

1. *Advanced cancer that cannot be removed by exploratory surgery;*

2. *Those with advanced cancer who have lost the indication for surgery;*

3. *Those who have metastasized or recurred in the near or long term after various cancer operations;*

4. *Liver metastasis, lung metastasis, brain metastasis of various advanced cancers or combined with cancerous pleural effusion and cancerous ascites;*

5. *All kinds of cancer resection surgery, exploration can only do gastrointestinal anastomosis or colostomy but not resection;*

6. *Patients who are not suitable for surgery, radiotherapy, chemotherapy, etc.*

XZ-C1, XZ-C4 anti-cancer Chinese medicine has been used in clinical practice for more than 10 years, and systematic observation has achieved obvious curative effect. No side effects have been seen after long-term use.

Clinical observations have proved that XZ-C1 and XZ-C4 anti-cancer Chinese medicine can comprehensively improve the quality of life of patients with advanced cancer, improve overall immunity, control cancer cell proliferation, and consolidate and enhance long-term efficacy. Oral and external application of XZ-C3 medicine has a good effect on softening and shrinking metastatic tumors on the body. With intervention or intubation drug pump treatment, it can protect the liver, kidney, bone marrow hematopoietic system and immune organs, and improve immunity.

3). XZ-C Anticancer Pain Relieving Ointment has good pain relief effect

Pain is a more obvious and painful symptom for patients with advanced cancer. General analgesics have little effect on cancer pain, and narcotic analgesics are addictive and dependent. XZ-C3 Anticancer Pain Relief Ointment has strong analgesic effect and lasts for a long time.

After 298 cases of clinical verification, the obvious effective rate is 78.0%, and the total effective rate is 95.3%. Repeated use has no obvious side effects, no addiction, and stable analgesic effects. It is an effective treatment method for cancer patients to relieve pain and improve the quality of life.

Through experimental research and clinical verification, our experience is:

Traditional Chinese medicine with Chinese characteristics has its unique advantages in tumor treatment, such as strong overall observation, outstanding conditioning effect, mild toxic and side effects, can relieve pain, relieve symptoms, significantly improve the quality of life of patients, and can modulate body immune function and overall disease resistance ability and improve treatment effect, or it can adjust the body's immune function and overall disease resistance, and improve the treatment effect.

4

Research on New Concepts and Methods of Cancer Metastasis Treatment

1) *__The research for the theory basis of the new cancer treatment__*

In 1985, the author surveyed more than 3000 cases of thoracic and abdominal surgeries made by him and found that cancer recurrence and metastasis are the key factors that affect postoperative curative effects.

It is necessary to do basic clinical research to prevent recurrence and metastasis

The author built a laboratory foe animal experiments

Made cancer-bearing animal model

New discoveries from the experimental researches

New Discovery 1:

Removal of thymus can make cancer-bearing animal model

New Discovery 2:
Immunosuppressant can weaken immunity to make the model

New Discovery 3:
Thymus atrophy with the development or evolvement of cancer

New Discovery 4:
Metastasis is related to immunity; weak immunity may accelerate metastasis
New Discovery 5:
Thymuses in the inoculated mice shrink progressively; those
without inoculation, there is no thymus atrophy.
When the tumor grows to the size of the finger tip, thymus is not continuous to shrink.
New Discovery 6:

Tumor can inhibit Thymus and cause the immune organs to shrink, therefore,
it is assumed that tumor can produce an unknown factor to inhibit Thymus,
which is called the factor of cancer inhibiting Thymus so far.

From the above experimental results, it can proposed:

While the tumor develop progressively,
1.The development or evolvement of tumors can make immune organs progressive atrophy;
2. Tumor decreases immunity progressively.

How to prevent TH atrophy?
How to promote immune surveillance?
The following research has been done in the laboratory

How to avoid thymus atrophy? How to avoid exhaustion of immunity?	How to prevent thymus atrophy? How to protect immune organs? How to strengthen immunity and avoid exhaustion of immunity

Immunologic reconstitution by adoptive immunity through transplantation of fetal liver, thymus and spleen cell	Look for the medicament that can prevent thymus atrophy and strengthen immunity from chinese medicine resource
The experimental results indicate that in the group of combined transplantation of S, T, L cells, the complete regression rate in near term is 40% and that of long term is 46.67%. Those with regression or disappeared can survive for a long time with good curative effects.	Then, we did screen experiments from 200chinese medication to look for the medication which can protect Thymus and increase immune function.
The aboveing experimental articles can not be published.	After 3 years of screen experiments: ①screening experiment by the rate of inhibiting tumors in vitro; ②screening experiment by the rate of inhibiting tumors in vivo of cancer-bearing animal model
It was to start to screen and look for natural medicament from traditional Chinese herbs through animal experiment.	

2) *The process of screening the anticancer medications*

XZ-C immune regulation and control anti-cancer and anti-metastasis Chinese medicine series products developed exclusively by XUZE

Aims:

Seek and screen anti-cancer and anti-metastatic Chinese herbal medicines from Chinese medicines

purpose:

It is to screen out "smart anticancer drugs" that are non-drug resistant, highly selective, non-toxic and side effects, and can be taken orally for a long time.

The route:

From experimental research to clinical verification, applied to clinical practice on the basis of successful animal experiments

The method:

To this end, we conducted animal experimental studies on 200 kinds of Chinese herbal medicines believed to have anti-cancer effects in traditional Chinese medicine to screen new anti-cancer and anti-metastatic drugs

Our laboratory has carried out the following experimental research on the cancer suppression rate of Chinese herbal medicine

(1) Our laboratory adopts the method of in vitro culturing of cancer cells to carry out the screening experiment of Chinese herbal medicines

(2) Our laboratory used EAC or S180 or H22 cancer cells to be inoculated to create cancer-bearing animal models, and to screen the anti-cancer rate of Chinese herbal medicine in cancer-bearing animals.

In vitro tumor inhibition screening test:

Culture cancer cells in vitro to observe the direct damage of drugs to cancer cells

In-test tube screening test:

Put crude drug products (500ug/ml) into the test tube for culturing cancer cells to observe the inhibitory effect on cancer cells

200 kinds of Chinese herbal medicines considered by traditional Chinese medicine to have anti-cancer effects, one by one in vitro screening test

Test and compare the control with fiber cell culture under the same conditions

Experimental results:

48 species have good tumor inhibition rates, and the other 152 (Chinese herbal medicines traditionally believed to have anti-cancer effects) have no obvious tumor inhibition effects

Test and compare the results of control experiments with fiber cell culture under the same conditions,

(2) Our laboratory used EAC or S180 or H22 cancer cells to be inoculated to create cancer-bearing animal models, and to screen the tumor inhibition rate of Chinese herbal medicine in cancer-bearing animals.

In vivo tumor suppression screening test:

Create animal models:

Mice inoculated with EAC or S180 or H22 cancer cells

Experiment grouping

In each batch of experiments, 240 mice were divided into 8 groups, 30 in each group. Group 7 was a blank control group, and group 8 was a control group with 5-FU or CTX.

After 24 hours of inoculation, each mouse was fed a certain amount of crude pharmaceutical powder, and the long-term feeding was used to observe the survival period and toxic and side effects, calculate the prolonged survival rate, and calculate the tumor inhibition rate.

Experimental results:

48 kinds of Chinese herbal medicines do have certain tumor inhibition rate. Among them, 26 have better anti-tumor effects. The 48 selected from this selection indeed have optimized combinations.

Repeated tumor inhibition rate experiments and immune experiments in cancer-bearing animal models

Finally, a preparation of XUZE China1-10 (XZ-C1-10), an immune-regulating anti-cancer traditional Chinese medicine with Chinese characteristics, was developed.

3) ***The clinical application of XZ-C immune regulation and control anticancer medications***

Clinical validation

A. *XZ-C immunomodulatory Chinese medicine is applied in clinical practice on the basis of experimental research*

B. *It was to perform clinical verification on the basis of successful animal experiments*

Establish an oncology clinic
It was to establish an anti-metastatic and recurrence scientific research team

↓

Keep outpatient medical records
Establish a regular follow-up observation system
Observe the long-term effect

↓

Observed on a large number of patients for 3-5 years
Even clinical observation for 8-10 years

↓

There are long-term follow-ups and evaluable treatments,

↓

The standard of efficacy is:

Good quality of life and long life span

↓

XZ-C immunomodulatory traditional Chinese medicine preparations have achieved remarkable curative effects after 25 years of application to a large number of patients with advanced cancer. Adopt XZ-C immune regulation to target cancer cells in metastasis, improve immune surveillance, and open up the third field of anti-cancer metastasis therapy.

↓

It can improve the quality of life of patients with advanced cancer, enhance immunity, improve immunity and regulatory capacity, increase the body's anti-cancer ability, increase appetite, increase physical strength, protect bone marrow, and enhance hematopoietic function.

Those who take the medicine for a longer period of time have recurrence after surgery, and the rate of metastasis is very small. Most of the patients who have metastasized or relapsed can stabilize the status quo without further metastasis.

Many patients with metastases from multiple organs can stabilize their condition, control metastasis, and prolong their survival significantly.

The data from clinical application verification

Clinical information:

From 1994 to November 2002, XZ-C immunomodulatory anti-cancer Chinese medicine was used to treat 4698 cases of stage III, IV or metastatic or recurrent cancer, including 3051 males and 1647 females. The oldest was 86 years old and the youngest was 11 years old. The entire group was diagnosed by histopathology or B-ultrasound, CT, MRI imaging, according to the International Anti-Cancer Alliance staging standards, all cases were patients with stage III or above.

Treatment results:

__The symptoms are improved, the quality of life is improved, and the survival period is prolonged.__

After 4277 patients with intermediate and advanced cancer had taken XZ-C immunoregulatory Chinese medicine for following-up more than 3 months, they showed various degrees of symptom improvement after taking the medicine, with an effective rate of 93.2%.

See Table 1 for general information, Table 2 for improving the quality of life of patients, Table 3 for changes in external application of swelling, and Table 4 for pain relief.

Table 1

General data of 4277 cases of recurrence and metastasis

		Liver cancer	Lung cancer	Stomach cancer	Esophagus Cardia Cancer	Rectal anal cancer	Colon cancer	Breast cancer	Pancreatic cancer
Number of cases		1021	752	668	624	328	442	368	74
Male: female		4:1	44:1	2.25:1	3.1:1	1:1	2.1:1	All women	32:1
Cancer foci	Primary	694 (68.8%)	699 (93.9%)						
	Metastasis	327 (31.2%)	53 (6.1%)						
Common places of transfers in this group		Lung Metastasis (2%) From Stomach (27.2%) From the esophagus Cardia Cancer (19.5%) From the rectum (31.2%)	Supraclavicular lymph node metastasis (11.6%) Brain metastasis (3.1%) Bone metastasis (4.6%)	Metastatic liver (23.8%) Lung metastasis (3%) Peritoneal metastasis (29.1%) Supraclavicular metastasis (6.1%)	Supraclavicular metastasis (13.1%) Liver metastasis (8.3%)	Recurrence rate (14.8%) Metastatic Liver (7.0%)	Metastatic liver (16.0%) Peritoneal Metastasis (6.0%)	Supraclavicular lymph node metastasis (175%) Axillary lymph node metastasis (15.0%) Bone metastasis (5.0%)	Metastatic liver (11.7%) etroperitoneal metastasis (39.1%)

Age	Peak age (years old) (%)							
	30-39 (76.2)	50-69 (71.6)	40-49 (73.4)	40-69 (80.4)	40-49 (75.2)	30-69 (88.0)	40-59 (55.9)	40-59 (70.0)
The Youngest (years old)	11	20	17	30	27	27	29	34
The oldest (years old)	86	80	77	77	78	76	80	68

Table 2

Observation of the curative effect of 4277 cases to improve the quality of life of patients with advanced cancer

	spirit	Appetite	Body Strengthen	Generally conditions improvement	Weight gain	Sleep better	Improve mobility Relief of restricted activity	Live independently walk as usual	Back to work Light work
Number of Improvement cases	4071	3986	2450	479	2938	1005	1038	3220	479

| % | 95.2 | 93.2 | 57.3 | 11.2 | 68.7 | 23.5 | 243 | 75.3 | 11.2 |

Table 3

Changes of 56 cases of metastatic nodules after external application of XZ-C ointment

| | Swollen supraclavicular lymph nodes in the neck | | | |
	disappear	Reduce 1/2	Turn soft	No change
Number of cases	12	22	14	8
	21.4	39.2	25.0	14.2
Total effective rate (%)	85.7			

Table 4

Pain relief after oral administration of XZ-C drug and external application of XZ-C anticancer pain relief ointment in 298 patients

| Symptoms | Pain | | | |
	Light reduced	significantly reduced	disappear	no effective
Number of cases %	52	139	93	14
	17.3	46.8	31.2	4.7
Total effective rate (%)	95.3			

In improving the quality of life (according to the Karnofsky score standard):
The average score is 50 points before taking the medicine, and 80 points after three months of taking the medicine, and some reach 90 or 100 points.

→

Survival analysis:

1. Outpatients are incomparable due to different disease stages and severity

2. Patients in this group are all above stage III, with metastasis and dysfunction of different tissues and organs.

3. According to previous statistics of such patients, the median survival time is about 6 months.

4. The longest cases in this group have reached 14 years, and the average survival time of the remaining cases is more than 1 year, for example:

One case of liver cancer recurrence after resection has been taking XZ-C for 14 years;

One case of liver cancer has been taking XZ-C for 10 and a half years;

3 cases of lung cancer couldn't be cut off, and they had been taking XZ-C medicine for 3 and a half years;

2 cases of remnant gastric cancer have been taking XZ-C medicine for 8 years;

3 cases of rectal cancer recurrence after surgery have taken XZ-C medicine for 3 years;

1 case of breast cancer metastasis to liver and ribs has been taking XZ-C medicine for 8 years;

One case of renal cancer recurrence after operation has taken XZ-C medicine for 9 and a half years.

These patients have undergone several long-term follow-up visits, picked up medications, and taken medications, and their condition is controlled in a stable state. The patients live with tumor for a long time. They have significantly prolonged the survival period.

Analysis of prolonged survival:

1. The typical cases of inoperable, radiotherapy, chemotherapy and XZ-C immunomodulatory anti-cancer Chinese medicine for more than 5 years are:

1. Di x x, left upper lung central lung cancer with left lung metastasis, served XZ-C1+4+7 for 5 years.

2. Huang xx, has been taking medication for esophageal cancer for 5 years

3. Huang xx, middle esophageal cancer has been taking medicine for 5 years

4. Huang xx, primary massive liver cancer has taken XZ-C medicine for 5 years

5. Qi xx, has taken XZ-C medicine for 5 years for primary liver cancer (see medical records for details)

2. The typical cases of using XZ-C immunomodulatory traditional Chinese medicine for 4 years are as follows:

1. It is x x, a tumor in the abdomen, which cannot be removed by exploratory surgery, has been taking XZ-C medicine for 4 years.

2. Recipe xx, pancreatic cancer cannot be detected by exploration, and I have been taking XZ-C medicine for 7 years.

3. Li xx, the primary massive liver cancer, cannot be detected by Tongji Hospital. He has been taking XZ-C medicine for 4 years.

4. Ke xx, primary liver cancer cannot be removed from the 301 hospital investigation, and has been taking XZ-C medicine for 5 years (see medical records for details)

5

The new model of Xu's (XZ-C) new concept
for anti-cancer metastasis treatment

Table
Cancer metastasis steps and treatment strategies

Transfer steps	Treatment strategy	XZ-C immunomodulation therapy
Primary cancer proliferation	Surgery, radiotherapy, chemotherapy	XZ-C1 inhibits cancer cells XZ-C4 Thymus protector XZ-C8 protects bone marrow and promotion of producing blood
Tumor angiogenesis	Inhibit angiogenesis	XZ-C2-TG anti-angiogenesis VA
Invasion of basement membrane	Anti-adhesion Anti-exercise Inhibit hydrolase activity	XZ-C2-CA Anti-adhesion VA XZ-C2-MD Anti-motion
Penetration into blood vessels or lymphatic vessels	Anti-adhesion Anti-exercise Inhibit hydrolase activity	X Z-C2-MD Anti-invasive blood vessel VA
In the blood of the circulatory system	Anti-platelet poly-anticoagulant response regulation BRM	XZ-C1-4 immune regulation and control XZ-C2-LM
Formation of tumor thrombus	Promoting blood circulation Removal of stasis Anti-thrombotic	XZ-C2-SAP cancer thrombus XZ-C1-4 immune regulation and control VA

Penetration out blood vessels or Pierce blood vessels	Anti-adhesion Anti-exercise Inhibit hydrolase activity	Z-C2-MD anti-invasion of blood vessels
Formation of metastases	Surgery, radiotherapy, chemotherapy	XZ-C1-4 immune regulation and control Z-C2-TG inhibits blood vessel growth
Metastatic lymph node	Fat-soluble agents	Brucea javanica emulsion

Printed in the United States
by Baker & Taylor Publisher Services